Advance Praise for
This Is How You Vagina

"Our bodies have been shrouded in shame and secrecy for far too long. Thank goodness Dr. Williams is here to pull back the curtain to help us to better understand and appreciate our bodies—all in the name of wellness, self-love, and pleasure."

—Jessica O'Reilly, PhD, sexologist, author of *The New Sex Bible*, and host of the podcast *Sex with Dr. Jess*

"Yes, we've lived with our vaginas for our entire lives, but I'm sure most women only have a cursory amount of knowledge about them. Dr. Nicole Williams successfully expands our knowledge of 'vajayjays' (and lays out the case why not to call them that). This is not a textbook; it's written with wit and logic and is easy to understand. She dispels trendy vaginal treatments and myths about what's 'good' and 'bad' for the vagina. Most importantly, once you have a better knowledge of this body part, you're equipped to treat it properly. Frankly, I think it's a book parents should have their daughters read as they begin puberty."

—Adrianna Hopkins, Emmy Award–winning news anchor and women's health advocate

"*This Is How You Vagina* is an excellent combination of history, science, and real talk from your bestie. Dr. Williams delivers tons of valuable information in an approachable way that will have you giggling while you are learning all about your lady bits."

—Sarah Deysach, owner of Early to Bed Sex Shop, Chicago, Illinois

"*This Is How You Vagina* is a refreshingly witty yet painstakingly accurate account of the female reproductive tract. As a practicing board certified gynecologist, I would recommend this book to every human with a vajayjay!"

—Ruth Arumala, DO, MPH, NCMP, FACOG

D1415152

THIS IS
HOW YOU
VAGINA

THIS IS HOW YOU VAGINA

All About Your Vajayjay and
Why You Probably Shouldn't Call It That

NICOLE WILLIAMS, MD, FACOG, FACS

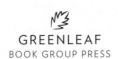

GREENLEAF
BOOK GROUP PRESS

Published by Greenleaf Book Group Press
Austin, Texas
www.gbgpress.com

Distributed by Greenleaf Book Group

For ordering information or special discounts for bulk purchases, please contact Greenleaf Book Group at PO Box 91869, Austin, TX 78709, 512.891.6100.

Design and composition by Greenleaf Book Group and Kim Lance
Cover design by Greenleaf Book Group and Kim Lance
Cover illustration of peach: iStock / Getty Images Plus / Dizolator
Author photo courtesy of Native Grind
Fig 1.4 courtesy of blueringmedia; Fig 2.3, 1884: purchases/Photographer: Marie-Lan Nguyen (2007); Fig 2.5 courtesy of Historical Collections & Services, Claude Moore Health Sciences Library, University of Virginia; Fig 12.1, The Great Wall of Vagina (panel 2 of 10) ©Jamie McCartney 2011

Publisher's Cataloging-in-Publication data is available.

Print ISBN: 978-1-62634-878-3

eBook ISBN: 978-1-62634-879-0

Part of the Tree Neutral® program, which offsets the number of trees consumed in the production and printing of this book by taking proactive steps, such as planting trees in direct proportion to the number of trees used: www.treeneutral.com

TreeNeutral

Printed in the United States of America on acid-free paper

21 22 23 24 25 26   10 9 8 7 6 5 4 3 2 1

First Edition

To my mother, who always believed.

My vagina's angry. It is. It's pissed off.
My vagina's furious and it needs to talk.
It needs to talk about all this shit.
It needs to talk to you. I mean, what's the deal—
An army of people out there thinking up ways to
torture my poor-ass, gentle, loving vagina.
Spending their days constructing psycho products
and nasty ideas to undermine my pussy.

Vagina Motherfuckers.

—THE VAGINA MONOLOGUES

What is a vagina other than me?

Is it sad, is it angry?

Does it bleed?

What is a vagina other than myself?

Is she happy does she experience joy?

Has she like me been put down

Ignored berated

Has she like me ever cried?

What is a vagina other than me?

Let's see . . .

Contents

Foreword

N ot long ago, I received a phone call from a younger physician, a gynecologist, who told me that she had written a book all about the vagina. She also told me that when she was a child in the 1990s she had held me up as a role model—someone to emulate, someone to learn from—and she wanted my critique of her work. Since we are members of the same sorority, Delta Sigma Theta, she thought I would be willing to, and I was. That physician was Dr. Nicole Williams. Her book, *This Is How you Vagina*, is an important addition to the realm of women's health information for the layperson.

Given my extensive experience and years in public health, having been the Director of Public Health for the State of Arkansas and the Surgeon General of the United States, I find it of the utmost importance that women be educated on their bodies—their function and even malfunction. Unfortunately, there is so much misinformation in the lay media that patients find it difficult to determine what is truth and what is fallacy. I believe that the way that Dr. Williams treats the subject, taking an historical bend and weaving it into physiology and present-day reality, is refreshing, fascinating, and informative.

All too often, we do not recognize each person's innate sexuality as being an important part of their humanity. This phenomenon starts at puberty and progresses into adulthood. And it is this nonrecognition that adds to the anxieties, particularly around sex, that women suffer from daily. When a natural part of our body can be seen or perceived as diseased and disgusting, it is no wonder that we are unable to fully embrace our bodies and ourselves in every way possible.

After having read *This Is How You Vagina*, I am heartened that the ability to confront and discuss difficult topics regarding women's sexuality and women's health has not been lost. This book is very clearly written and provides an abundance of useful information for adolescents, childbearing age women, and mature or elderly women. The information is comprehensive, concrete, and accurate and vital for women to make informed decisions about their sexual and reproductive health. It is an excellent resource for women who have questions about their bodies and are perhaps too embarrassed to ask. Dr. Williams is a fresh new voice in the debate on women's health, and it is my sincere hope that many others will read, listen, and join in the conversation.

—**M. Joycelyn Elders, M.D.**
former Surgeon General of the United States of America
Professor Emerita at the University of Arkansas School of Medicine
author of *From Sharecropper's Daughter to
Surgeon General of the United States of America*

Introduction

Please allow me to introduce myself. My name is Dr. Nicole Williams, and I am a gynecologist. I am also female. The combination of my own vagina experience paired with scientific and anatomical knowledge gives me the insight to be able to help you, my fellow vagina owners, learn to treat yours right.

Beginning in middle school, my friends and I started to hear the rumors. We're not quite sure exactly where or how they started, but they seemed to materialize sometime after eighth grade. We had this mysterious body part that smelled bad. You couldn't see it very well. It got hairy. It bled practically every month, and to top it all off, there was discharge. Ugh. It was no wonder that when I went to medical school, I was excited to learn the truth about my vagina, the truth about the form and function of our anatomy and physiology. But no—that didn't happen. In graduate school, I received practically the same canned knowledge I could have gotten from Judy Blume.

In my work today as a gynecologist, the most common complaints and issues my patients come to me with were utterly absent from my medical school studies—which were conservative, unempowering, and downright boring. When I graduated, I could rattle off each of the pro-hormones, enzymes, molecules, and other minute interactions involved in the function of the vagina and its parts, but her true nature did not reveal herself to me until years later. After completing my residency in obstetrics and gynecology, I started really talking to patients and learning about their concerns. I realized that their perceptions of their own vaginas were colored by those same middle school rumors that I had heard growing up.

I am the daughter of teachers, and I have always understood the value of a proper education and the dangers of misinformation. It is important that we as vagina owners understand her fully, embrace her in all her glory, and love her as she is. And that is what I aim to help you do.

So, what is the vagina? The number of words for vagina, is honestly, astounding:

beaver	cunt	glory hole
concha	hole	taco
bitch	bearded clam	bizcocho
box	crack	pepita
cherry	fanny	bucketpucha
gash	meat curtains	snooch
merkin	cookie	mossy cleft
muff	quim	bean
pudenda	honey pot	love canal
toto	guayabo	peach
punani	maneater	carpet
puss	yoni	kitty
pussy	minge	poontang
slit	vag	crica
la cosa loca	camel toe	mico
slut	trim	cha-cha
vajayjay	putz	la bomba
cunny	fur burger	veriga
snatch	grumble	nether regions
twat	papaya	squeezebox
sperm sucker	mound	

This list is *far* from exhaustive. And, as there are innumerable names for the vagina, there are also endless myths and misinformation about this most fascinating organ. Did you know it was once thought that the vagina was simply an inside-out penis? That there were ancient cultures who thought that some vaginas actually had biting teeth? I would hazard to say that some of these beliefs came from the whole biblical Adam's rib/fallen Eve thing, with women being simply a version of man or having body parts that could literally bite men. (Note that one of the slang terms for vagina is *maneater*.)

Many of my patients, both young and old, have presented to me on various occasions some of their vagina misinterpretations as fact. When I see a new patient, I tell them to think of me like a plumber or a priest and tell me all. And they do. I've heard that if you squat over a steaming pot of herbs, your period symptoms will get better and your vagina will be detoxified. I've been told that little green eggs can help regulate pH. I've had patients tell me they douche or pee after sex so they won't get pregnant or get a UTI. (You don't have to do either of these.)

I was motivated to write this book to dispel the cacophony of misinformation from nearly everywhere these days, including the internet, magazines, peers, and even in some schools, about this most important functioning organ, the vagina. I distinctly recall participating in a seminar where the educator advocated for the daily use of panty liners, sleeping in underwear, and not using tampons to an audience of rapt 10- to 12-year-olds, curious and attentive. As opposed to waging an outright war (though I wanted to), I kept my cool and advised that each girl talk to her pediatrician. If this is the type of thinking that is being disseminated to preteens today, it's no wonder my adult patients are confused! Listening to my patients ask me the same questions every day, over and over again, got me thinking: How can I best inform my patients about their wonderful vaginas without lecturing them?

I pored over hundreds of articles, books, and websites, many of which were either overly technical or overly simplified, and I thought, *Let's make this better*. How can I make the vagina understandable and accessible, without talking down to my (very intelligent) patients? How can I write a book that you can read cover to cover, explaining with science but not putting you to sleep? Here is my effort—hope it worked!

1

Greetings, I'm Your Vagina

Consider me your friendly neighborhood vagina doctor.

—ME

The vagina is a fascinating organ. It is not just a "hole" or some chasm or abyss of never-ending space. You can't get lost in there. It is a real, functioning organ, with receptors and the means to communicate with its environment unlike any other. It serves a very particular purpose, a unique one in humanity. It serves as both a sexual and functional organ, able to give us indescribable pleasure during sex and allowing enough stretch for the birth of a human child. It is a truly spectacular entity in that it actually works quite well in both capacities. I am always amazed at how it can give way to a six-pound baby, yet still maintain an erogenous zone capable of facilitating mind-blowing orgasms! What other organ in all the world can do such a thing? She is special. And just over half the world has one.

WHAT DOES SHE LOOK LIKE?

You may have already noticed, but in this book, we will use the term *vagina* to represent the entirety of female genitalia, given that many don't recognize or understand the term *vulva*. The vagina is actually the part of the female genitalia that is inside a women's body, and the vulva includes those parts that exist on the outside of the body. But, for clarity's sake, we will refer to the whole of female genitalia collectively as the vagina.

Although there is wide anatomical variation, the length of the unaroused vagina of a woman of childbearing age is about 2.5 to 3 inches across the front, and 3.5 inches long across the rear. She starts at the cervix (the bottom of the uterus) and ends at the hymen or introitus (the opening of the vagina). The opening of the vagina is somewhat smaller in diameter than the top, near the cervix.

If you are looking at the vagina from the top down, you can see there is a series of ligaments and fascia that hold her in place. The support system of the vaginal walls causes the opening of the vagina to often look like an H shape at the opening. This turns into a convex smiley-face shape close to the top near the uterus, like this:

FIG. 1.1

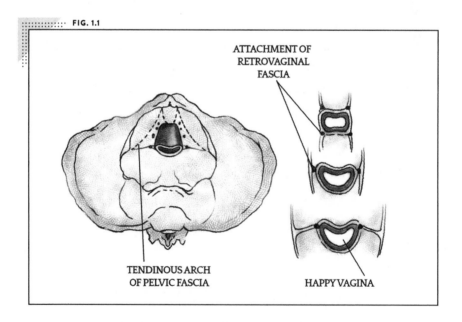

SEE THE BOTTOM RIGHT IMAGE? NOW THAT'S A HAPPY VAGINA!

Although there have been plenty of studies about the sizes and shapes of male genitalia, there have been very few for women. However, according to research we do have, a few MRI studies from the late 1990s and early to mid-2000s, the vagina can take a few different internal shapes. All of these shapes are *normal* anatomical variations of each other:

- Parallel-sided (H shape)
- Heart-shaped
- Conical
- Pumpkin seed
- Slug-shaped

FIG. 1.2

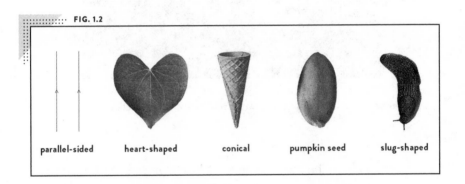

parallel-sided   heart-shaped   conical   pumpkin seed   slug-shaped

ILLUSTRATION OF THE NORMAL ANATOMICAL VAGINA SHAPES.
VARIATIONS OF THESE TYPES ARE ALSO NORMAL.

Lengthwise, the vagina generally follows a gentle, sloping angle that leads to the uterus. This canal is where your tampon or menstrual cup is held in place, and the lack of direct nerve endings (meaning no clitoral nerve parts) in this part of the vagina is why you can't feel things once they have been properly placed.

With arousal, the vagina can expand in both length and width in order to accommodate nearly any penis. In fact, the vagina can expand up to 200 percent during sexual arousal. (So no, he's never "too big" for you.)

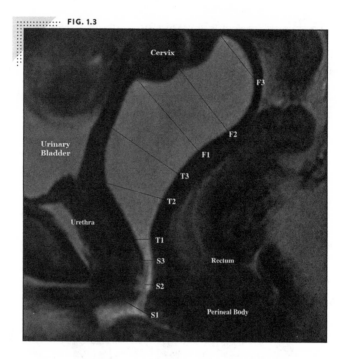

FIG. 1.3

MRI OF THE VAGINA FROM A LATERAL VIEW. SEE HOW THE DIAMETER CHANGES?

According to the MRI studies mentioned above, the conical vagina shape seems to be the most common. Most vaginas have three generalized zones. The first is more like a sphincter; this is where you find muscular support and where those muscles can spasm and cause pain during sex. The second zone is a wedge-shaped transitional zone, and the third is deeper and more expanded, where the vagina angles to meet the uterus.

WHERE IS SHE, ANYWAY?

The vagina is located between the openings of your urethra and anus, and she is usually the most prominent of those three, anatomically speaking. To see the vagina, hold a mirror there (it may be easiest to lie on your back to do this) and open the labia with your fingers. The urethra (the opening for urine) is also between these labia. It is a slit-like opening positioned above the vagina.

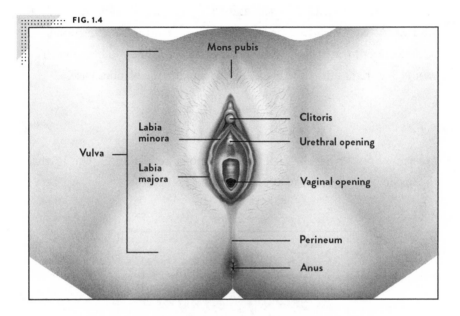

FIG. 1.4

Mons pubis

Clitoris

Labia
minora — Urethral opening

Vulva —

Labia
majora — Vaginal opening

Perineum

Anus

ANATOMY OF THE FEMALE EXTERNAL GENITALIA.

Externally, you may see little pink fingerlike projections around the opening of your vagina. This is *normal*. If you've already had sex, this is the remnant of the hymen, which partially covered the vaginal opening until some type of penetration may have caused it to break. If the hymen is still intact, you most likely will not be able to fully see the opening, but you may see the pink membrane of the hymen at the bottom of the vagina. It's OK to touch it (you should!)—you can't hurt it with just a finger. In fact, even if you've never had sex, it may already have a little tear, and this is completely OK. In a little over 50 percent of young women, the hymen has already been torn before engaging in penetrative sex the first time.

While you're looking, check out your perineum. That's the area between your vagina and anus. Squeeze the muscles surrounding the area a few times.

It's like making a fist with your vagina. Watch what happens. Cool, right? Now that's power! This is what's known as a Kegel exercise.

The very small hole you see at the top, the urethra, is where urine is released. It's pretty hard to see, and I have had more than one medical student try to put a catheter in the vagina to drain urine, so if you don't see it, that's OK. If you urinate, then you can safely assume you have one. The vagina lives right under the bladder and supports the bladder base.

WHAT'S SHE MADE OF?

Let's move on to what the vagina looks like on a cellular level. This is what the inside of a vagina looks like under a microscope:

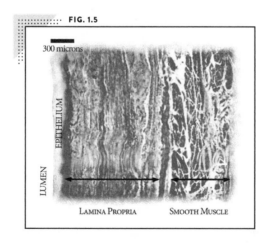

FIG. 1.5

300 microns

EPITHELIUM

LUMEN

LAMINA PROPRIA   SMOOTH MUSCLE

THE VAGINA AS SEEN UNDER A MICROSCOPE IN CROSS SECTION. NOTICE THE DISTINCT LAYERS
BETWEEN THE MUCOSA, THE TISSUE UNDERNEATH, AND THE LAYERS OF MUSCLE.

Inside our body, the vagina is a fibromuscular tube—*muscular* being the key part of that term. This makes sense for a few reasons: One, muscles allow for involuntary vaginal contractions post-orgasm, which can help keep semen inside and close to the top of the vagina so sperm can easily gain access to the uterus through the cervix for fertilization. Two, muscles can help with expansion and contraction of the vagina during and after childbirth.

The *epithelium* lines the opening, or *lumen,* of the vagina. It is covered by *epithelial,* or outer, cells. These types of cells are very similar to other mucous membranes, such as the mouth or rectum, and similar in color (reddish-pink). The epithelium serves to protect, expand, and provide moisture. When supported by estrogen, it makes the vagina scrunch into folds called *rugae,* which allows for expansion and lubrication and aids in sexual pleasure, allowing a penis to move freely in and out.

The *lamina propria* is rich in elastic fibers. This is the portion of the vagina that allows for stretching to accommodate nearly any sized penis during arousal and aids in expansion for childbirth.

The smooth muscle layer is inside the lamina propria. Unlike a biceps or a triceps muscle, which have striated or straight fibers, smooth muscle is more disordered, meaning the muscle fibers go in many different directions. This special construct is quite helpful in overall vaginal function. In fact, the uterus is also made up of smooth muscle; the bladder has some too. In addition, tiny bits of smooth muscle surround the intestines to move food and major blood vessels to move blood. This particular type of muscle maintains what's called a *resting tone* to keep the shape of hollow organs such as the uterus, vagina, and bladder. When smooth muscle contracts, it is an involuntary movement triggered by nerve impulses that travel to the smooth muscle tissue (like that after an orgasm). The disorderly arrangement of cells within smooth muscle tissue allows for contraction and relaxation with great elasticity; this is especially useful for an organ that often must double in size over the course of minutes or hours.

Your vagina also contains collagen, a special type of protein. While there are about twenty-eight different types of collagen found in the human body, your vagina contains what is called *fibrillar collagen,* which comes in different types. Type I fibrillar collagen is the most common type of collagen in the human body and helps to provide the three-dimensional framework that builds our bodies (including our vaginas). While your vagina contains mainly type III, another fibrillar collagen that forms smaller, more flexible, distensible tissue, your vagina also contains a fair amount of type I collagen. To explain how strong your vagina is, know that type I collagen has a greater tensile strength than steel. Try mentioning that at your next dinner party.

FIG. 1.6

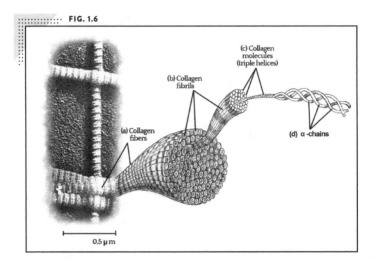

COLLAGEN: THE BUILDING BLOCK OF YOUR VAGINA (AND MOST EVERYTHING ELSE IN YOUR BODY). SEE HOW DENSELY PACKED THE FIBERS ARE?

HOW DOES SHE LUBRICATE?

Now that we know what your vagina is made of, let's delve a little deeper into how she works. Oftentimes, my patients' biggest complaint is vaginal discharge. Fortunately, most discharge is normal. Normal vaginal fluid is primarily composed of water, protein, and (generally healthy) bacteria, primarily *Lactobacilli*.[1]

Where does this water come from? It comes from what's called a *transudate*. What is a transudate? It's a filtrate of blood that allows for a bit of leakage of water and protein through the tissue and into the vagina, therefore keeping a supply of moisture that can ebb and flow according to many factors, sexual stimulation included.

WHAT ABOUT BACTERIA?

You may be thinking, "Eww," but I say not "Eww," but "Ahh!" Bacteria are everywhere on and inside our bodies. They are found in our mouths, intestines, skin, and all mucous membranes. The vagina is no exception, and for the most part, these bacteria are symbiotic and overall quite helpful. The types of bacteria vary depending on location. The predominant bacteria in the vagina is called *Lactobacilli*.[2] Interestingly, *Lactobacilli* is also found in a healthy intestinal tract. Coincidence? I think not. Healthy gut, healthy vagina!

Other bacteria commonly identified in the normal vaginal microbiome include several *Staphylococcus* species along with *Ureaplasma, Corynebacterium, Streptococcus, Peptostreptococcus, Gardnerella, Bacteroides, Mycoplasma, Enterococcus, Escherichia, Veillonella, Bifidobacterium,* and *Candida.* Yes, *Candida!* You might assume that the presence of any *Candida* means you have a yeast infection, but it's actually OK if you have a few strains of it; it's when the balance of bacteria is disturbed that problems can occur.

The vagina is colonized with bacteria within hours of a baby girl's birth and remains as such until death. At puberty, vaginal estrogen levels increase; this results in an increase in *Lactobacilli. Lactobacilli* sticks to the vaginal walls to help keep her healthy and promote healthy sexual function. It is a friendly type of bacteria that works to tamp down harmful bacterial invaders in the vagina by producing antimicrobial compounds such as hydrogen peroxide and lactic acid. This also lowers the vaginal pH, which helps kill unhealthy sperm, only allowing the best and strongest through her gates. See how beautifully this works?[3]

BUT WHAT ABOUT THE CLITORIS?

Now that we have an inkling of vaginal anatomy, the clitoris deserves an anatomy and physiology lesson all by herself. Georg Ludwig Kobelt, a 19th-century German anatomist, was possibly the first who thought so. In his *Die männlichen und weiblichen Wollust-Organe des Menschen und einiger*

Säugetiere (*The Male and Female Organs of Sexual Arousal in Man and Some Other Mammals*) published in 1844, he featured the first comprehensive anatomical dissection and drawing of the anatomy of the clitoris known to date. For comparison, the first version of *Gray's Anatomy*, published in the United States in 1859, depicted the female anatomy without the clitoris at all. It took more than a hundred years to get a detailed picture of the organ and learn that there is much more to the clitoris than meets the eye. Even though the clitoris was pictured in later versions of anatomy books, we didn't have a complete picture of the organ until the 1990s, with the help of MRI. MRI allowed us to visualize living women as opposed to cadavers to attempt to fully understand this overlooked and understudied neurovascular bundle. Since then, much more has been discovered about the complexity of the organ and its relationship to the vagina and urethra. In fact, modern (since the early 2000s) anatomy books have had to be rewritten to underscore and emphasize the marvelously complicated clitoris.

First of all, the clitoris is much larger than most of us think. You might imagine this tiny little button just barely peeking out from under its protective hood, but that is literally just the tip of the iceberg. The clitoris travels far and wide in the vaginal complex.

FIG. 1.7

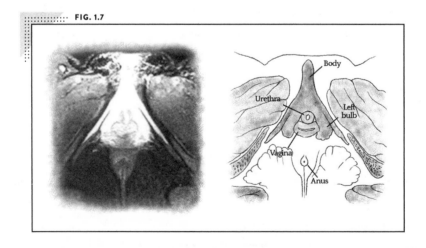

THE CLITORIS AS SEEN ON MRI. IT'S MUCH LARGER THAN YOU THINK!

Imagine you are looking at a woman from her feet with her lying on her back. The clitoris sits immediately above the opening of the vagina. You may notice that the clitoris looks fairly similar to the glans and body of the penis.

The names are similar because they are developmentally similar. The glans, crura, and bulb essentially match male anatomy, except in one thing: the nerves. The female clitoris has twice as many nerve endings as the penis. The nerves of the clitoris come from where all our nerves do: the spinal cord. So let's follow the nerves. From the very bottom of your tailbone comes the pudendal nerve. That nerve branches out to feed everything in the lower half of your body. The clitoral and peroneal neurovascular bundles are where you find the nerve endings, paired terminations of the pudendal neurovascular bundles. However, the branch that forms the clitoris seems to be different. There is an intimate connection between the nerves and the surrounding erectile tissue (tissue capable of behavior similar to an erection) called the bulbs. These bulbs are spongy in character and are connected to the urethra, crura, and corpora to form what is called the root of the clitoris.

Interestingly, we have yet to determine the exact function of the bulbs in urethral and sexual function. What we do know through MRI is that the bulbs seen on either side of the urethra continue to the front portion of the urethra and meet in the middle. It took a while, but anatomy doctors finally agreed that these bulbs are not actually part of the urethra but are related to the clitoris. Where the bulbs and body meet at the top of the vagina might provide evidence of the G-spot.

Now that we know a bit more about the basic anatomy and physiology of the vagina, let's take a look at how she is represented in history.

DID YOU KNOW?

Both sharks and vaginas make the same lubricant. It's called *squalene*.

2

Vaginas: A Brief History

I've tried everything! Garlic, yogurt, everything!

—R. M., AGE 33

I n order to gain a full understanding of how we in modern society have come to understand the vagina, let's explore the customs of some ancient cultures. One of the earliest records of gynecological practices was found in 1889, when a papyrus was discovered near the modern-day Egyptian town of El Lahun. The so-called Kahun Gynecological Papyrus is one of the largest manuscripts dating from the late Middle Kingdom (1850–1700 BCE) of the ancient Egyptian empire. The papyrus describes various conditions, remedies, and techniques, from sore limbs and heavy bleeding to predicting the gender of a baby before it was born. None of these remedies have been demonstrated to be effective, but having some insight into early theories about women's health and how our own beliefs have been formed is interesting. Although the ancient Egyptians were well known for their study of the underworld, it appears their study of the world-down-under was lacking.

The ancient Egyptians seemed to think that any problem a woman experienced was somehow related to her womb. Unfortunately, this is an attitude that persists to this day. If a woman is angry, it must be because she has PMS. It's as if women are not allowed to become upset by the usual life occurrences that would make anyone—male or female or nonbinary— angry. But the Ancient Egyptians may have taken this idea a little far.

THE MIGRATING WOMB

In ancient Egypt, nearly all women's maladies were attributed to vaginal discharge or the "migrating womb." The theory of the migrating womb is this: When a woman had any problem, whether it be in the head, the foot, or anywhere in between, it was believed that the uterus had traveled to that spot to cause her turmoil.

Take this example from the Kahun Papyrus, detailing the diagnosis and treatment of a woman with sore eyes or neck:

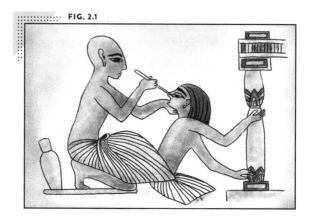

FIG. 2.1

**EXAMINATION OF A WOMAN WHOSE EYES ARE ACHING UNTIL SHE
CANNOT SEE, ON TOP OF ACHES IN HER NECK.**

*You should say of it "it is discharges of the womb in her eyes."
You should treat it by fumigating her with incense and fresh oil,
fumigating her womb with it, and fumigating her eyes with
goose leg fat. You should have her eat a fresh ass liver.*[1]

In this instance, the womb (uterus) made its way to the woman's eyes to make the discharge, and as treatment she was prescribed vaginal steaming and eating an ass's liver. Note that this is the earliest evidence of vaginal steaming. I'm certainly glad ass's liver didn't catch on.

FIG. 2.2

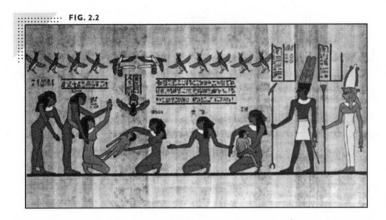

THIS PAPYRUS DEPICTS CHILDBIRTH WITH HELP FROM OTHER WOMEN AND THE GODS.

Here is an ancient treatment for a urinary tract infection. Again, nearly all women's maladies were attributed to vaginal discharge or the "migrating womb." Here is a loose translation from the Kahun Gynecological Papyrus:

> *Examination of a woman aching in her urine . . .*
> *You should say of it "it is discharges of the womb."*
> *You should treat it with beans, plant and parts of the gyw plant.*
> *Grind, refine with a jar of beer. Boil, drink on four mornings.*
> *She spends one day and night fasting, the morning after drink of the same.*
> *She spends one day fasting until the arrival of breakfast time.*

The ancient Greeks also adopted the Egyptians' "discharges" of the womb concept and characterized the womb as being an entirely separate entity, apart from the woman herself. It was free to leave its normal place and travel anywhere in the woman's body. The result is a condition called *hysteria* from the Greek *hystera*, or womb, that attributed all women's concerns to the uterus going awry. According to a treatise by Aretaeus of Cappadocia, the womb was an animal!

> *In women, in the hollow of the body below the ribcage, lies the womb. It is very much like an independent animal within the body for it moves around of its own accord and is quite erratic. Furthermore, it likes fragrant smells and moves toward them, but it dislikes foul odors and moves away from them . . . When it suddenly moves upward [i.e., toward a fragrant smell] and remains there for a long time and presses on the intestines, the woman chokes, in the manner of an epileptic . . .*[2]

Of course, hysteria primarily affected women who did not fill what was thought to be the prescribed social role of women. Those who did not become pregnant were lesbians; those who lived some nontraditional life-style seemed to have uteri that liked to wander about much more than those who got pregnant and lived a more conventional lifestyle.[3]

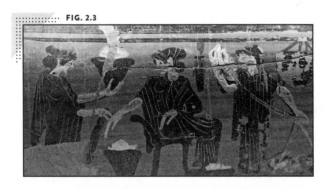

FIG. 2.3

WOMEN DEPICTED IN THE GREEK GYNACEUM,
WOMEN'S QUARTERS OF THE HOUSE, CIRCA 500 BC.

Apparently, the uterus is attracted to fragrant smells, can induce choking and seizures, and is overall a miserable organ to possess. A woman who had a seizure disorder was therefore hysterical because her uterus was out of order. The concept of the migrating womb migrated more than five hundred years through time, and even today, when we call women "hysterical" it implies that their emotions are tied to their reproductive functioning.

Many of the ancient cures for women involved using fragrances and other materials to lure the animalistic uterus back into place. Bad odors such as burnt linen, pitch, and burnt leather were given to the poor woman to smell, while sweet smells like chamomile and musk oils were applied to the vagina. Luckily, with modern science and our understanding of anatomy, today's gynecologists don't feel the need to lure uteruses back where they are supposed to be, because we know they never left.

THEY PUT WHAT IN WHERE?

Besides the migrating womb theory, ancient Egyptians came up with a host of cures for all kinds of vaginal maladies, including bacterial vaginosis and yeast infections. The Ebers Papyrus from 1550 BCE was a treatise on various herbs and their uses. If a patient complained of having vaginal discharge, it recommended helping the woman by crushing up earth from the Nile with honey and galena, putting it inside a wad of linen, and leaving it inside her. Please do not try this at home.[4]

Vaginal bleeding was also treated in an interesting way. Here is an excerpt from the Kahun Papyrus:

> *Examination of a woman bleeding . . . human mother,*
> *aching in her head, her mouth and the palm of her hand.*
> *You should treat it by smearing for her ground and placing on it*
> *[the vagina] dregs of sweet beer. [If] nothing emerges for her,*
> *you should place dates in . . . causing her to sit on it . . .*

Placing dregs of sweet beer near the vagina may not have helped a woman's bleeding problem, but it could cause a heck of a yeast infection![5]

Placing items in the vagina for various purposes has apparently always been done. You might have heard about the use of garlic in the vagina as a treatment for yeast infections (that doesn't work). According to the Ebers Papyrus, the ancient Egyptians recommended placing an onion bulb into a woman's vagina overnight to increase fertility. If you could smell onion on her breath in the morning, she was considered fertile. While we will focus later on why inserting vegetables into your vagina is highly ineffective, it is fascinating to me that this has been going on for literally millennia.

The Egyptians weren't *all* wrong, by the way. They did devise various contraceptives, some of which have been proven somewhat effective, and all of which had to be inserted into the vagina. Inserts made of sour milk, honey with a pinch of natron, or acacia gum were commonly used.[6]

Interestingly, acacia gum has been demonstrated to work, at least to a certain extent. It has a spermicidal effect, which comes from our happy bacteria friend *Lactobacilli*. Acacia gum is fermented by the bacteria into lactic acid, which serves as a mild spermicide. Of course, its effectiveness could not have been quite as good as what we have access to today, but if you were a female in ancient times, this was cutting edge.[7]

Another contraceptive that has been documented by the Egyptians is crocodile dung. Used around 1800 BCE, the fecal matter was mixed with dough and sprinkled onto and inserted into the vagina. It appears to have worked more similarly to a diaphragm, by blocking the entry of sperm into the womb proper.

Other ancient cultures from India and the Middle East used elephant dung for a similar purpose. But since dung is slightly alkaline, and sperm are as well, theoretically they would thrive in the naturally acidic environment of the vagina. Seems to be not exactly the most effective form of birth control.

Birth control appeared to be the primary reason to put something in one's vagina, and the insertion of items continued into the time of the Greeks. In fact, a fairly effective form of birth control was found in the fruit of the pomegranate (*punica granatum*). This insert, similar to acacia gum, has roots in science. The peel of the pomegranate has been shown to decrease fertility in lab rats. A recipe from the Greek physician Soranus in the 2nd century CE involves the use of pomegranate peel or rind inserted into the vagina. Ancient lore discusses eating the pomegranate seeds themselves,[8] and the use of the pomegranate as an abortifacient and contraceptive has also been described in ancient Indian texts.

Although many of these ancient ideas have been completely debunked, it is not surprising how these basic thoughts and teachings about the vagina have persisted through the centuries and pervaded and invaded even our modern thinking.

EARLY EXAMINATIONS

Let's imagine it's the 12th century in southern Italy. You are a wealthy merchant's wife, and you wake up one day with a rash all over your body, a headache, and a sore throat. Luckily, because of your status, you have access to some of the most advanced care available at the time. You visit the local physician, and immediately he tells you that your uterus has migrated to your throat. To cure you, he might prescribe baths, tampons of herbs, or even leeches (oh, hell no).

One interesting thing to note about these long ago doctor visits is that the physicians who treated female patients were most likely male and had never actually touched a living female or ever examined her genitals in a medical capacity. Most practitioners who treated women used a compendium text from southern Italy called *On the Diseases of Women*, which oddly enough is thought to have been produced by a woman, a mysterious figure known as Trotula. Although mysteries and misconceptions abounded, some practitioners had begun to examine women, a novel concept then, to learn more about how the vagina actually works. Trotula's work described the use of acacia and pomegranate, demonstrating what had been proven to be useful in the past centuries was learned and utilized. Unfortunately, many of these pioneer women in medicine have been lost to history, and the vagina and her cohorts remained a mystery until nearly modern times.

The 19th century brought with it some strange customs. The idea of utilizing so-called "pelvic massage" developed during this time. This is not the modern-day pelvic floor physical therapy that has been studied to be useful. It was instead a system of both external and internal manipulation purported to cure a variety of conditions such as heavy bleeding, miscarriage, ovarian cysts, enlargement of the uterus, and prolapse of the genital organs.

Dr. Thure Brandt began treating women with his method of pelvic massage in 1861. The first descriptions of the Brandt method were published in the *New York Medical Journal* in 1876. His technique entailed some stretching and application of pressure, which is fine, but it's upon the insertion of a finger that things get weird. A point-by-point instruction guide with seven steps of internal massage was published in 1898 by one of Brandt's followers, Dr. Robert Ziegenspeck, in his book *Massage Treatment (Thure Brandt) in Diseases of Women: For Practitioners.* Incredibly detailed and occasionally graphic, it is a wonder it was published:

1. The patient's dress is not removed, not even thrown back, but merely opened around the waist. The corset likewise is loosened, so that no hook or band may interfere. The chemise is then pulled up so far that the hand can be placed upon the bare abdomen; the abdomen itself, however, is not uncovered.

2. The finger to be introduced into the vagina, from underneath the knee of the side corresponding to the hand employed, can also be advanced beneath the dress towards the vaginal orifice without the knees being separated.

3. Only one finger is introduced under all circumstances—preferably the forefinger, except in ventro-vaginal-rectal palpation, where the forefinger is inserted into the rectum and the thumb into the vagina.

4. The hand laid upon the abdomen feels its way towards the finger in the vagina, not with uniform pressure, but penetrating deeper and deeper by means of gentle circular massage movements.

5. The examiner, seated upon a chair at the end of a couch, takes the corner of the latter between his separated knees.

6. Only a low bench, couch, or so-called plinth is used and no examining chair or table.

7. The unemployed fingers are not flexed (examination with closed hand) but rest loosely extended in the groove between the nates (examination with open hand).

Yes, this was published in an actual medical text. Using "gentle circular massage movements" was considered medical treatment during the Victorian age. While some of these treatments were recommended to persist for fifteen minutes, they advised practitioners to avoid producing "sexual irritation" (meaning sexual arousal). If advice was given against producing arousal, we can safely infer that sexual "irritation" must have occurred quite commonly. Of course, all of these actions occurred without ever disrobing the patient, with the examiner's hand searching beneath the patient's skirts.[9]

Have you ever wondered why your doctor puts a sheet over your bottom half during your gynecologic exam, and once you're lying down you usually can't see what they're doing or their faces when they're doing it? Here you can credit 19th-century medicine. The voluminous skirts worn by women of that day provided for convenient cover and kept physician-patient contact to a minimum. Remember, during that time, examiners hardly ever (meaning never) actually looked at their patients' vaginas and often avoided any eye contact when performing a manual exam. Unfortunately, with the sensibilities of 19th-century humans, there was a need to separate the woman herself from the examination of her body, since women were considered the "weaker sex." Married women were considered the property of their husbands and absolutely unequal to men. It is likely that this unequal treatment translated to their reproductive organs and the examination thereof. What I was told in medical school was that we used a sheet to protect "patient modesty," quite reminiscent of the Victorian attitude of needing to "protect" the female patient. Even though I still use a sheet when performing these exams, I make a little bend in the sheet so you can see my face and I can see you—primarily as a sign of respect.

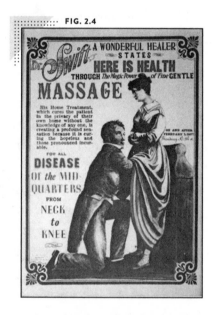

FIG. 2.4

NOTICE THE LACK OF EYE CONTACT BETWEEN PATIENT AND EXAMINER. ALSO, HOW COULD HE SEE WHAT HE WAS DOING?

As medicine was developing, there was a need for people to learn from one another, and learning the skills of gynecology was no exception. In the late 18th and into the 19th centuries, the operating room was literally a theater. (I've been to some places in the world where they still call it that, without the stadium seats, of course.) The surgeons were the stars, and the patients mere props in the show. The rooms were set up like amphitheaters, or theaters-in-the-round, with observers peering from above down into the operating space. These crowded, poorly lit places were where the beginnings of modern surgery were born. There, visionary physicians such as Dr. James Lister recognized the existence of germs and the importance of cleaning the hands, and William Stewart Halsted pioneered the surgical treatment of a dangerous obstetric condition, placenta previa. Although early surgeons did not separate themselves from their patients' faces, my theory is that today we set up the sterile sheet and the anesthesiologist makes a little tent separating the patient's head and shoulders from the rest of the body to "protect patient modesty." Perhaps these are merely the vestiges of history.

THE ORIGINS OF THE VAGINAL SPECULUM

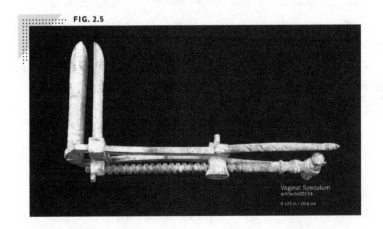

FIG. 2.5

Vaginal Speculum
artifacts00154

8.125 in / 20.6 cm

AN ANCIENT VAGINAL SPECULUM WHICH LOOKS REMARKABLY SIMILAR TO WHAT WE USE TODAY.

Just the mere mention of the word *speculum* may make you want to perform a Kegel, but this most dreaded and useful of devices got its start thousands of years ago. One of the reasons why the design hasn't changed in all that time is simple: It's really good at doing what it's supposed to do. Properly inserted, it reveals the only internal organ you can see without cutting, the cervix. The first known speculum was used in ancient Rome around the year 97 CE (or 79 CE depending on which article you reference), and it looks remarkably similar to the one used today, with the exception of a rather fascinating-looking corkscrew to hold it open. Unfortunately, this object was found near Pompeii, and so no paper documentation has been discovered to test these early physicians' knowledge.

I find it strange that as history progresses, we move from the curiosity of the female genitalia exhibited in ancient Rome to the blind skirt-reaching of the Victorian age. However, I would like to introduce another pioneering female physician into the mix who could have changed everything in the Victorian age, had she been around: Frenchwoman Madame Marie Anne Boivin. Born in 1773, she attended midwifery school at the Hôtel-Dieu in the Hospice de la Maternité, a well-known teaching hospital in Paris. A prolific medical writer and researcher, she was one of the first to use a stethoscope to listen to the fetal heart and also developed a way to measure the birth canal. Her most important invention from a vagina standpoint, however, is that of the modern-day vaginal speculum. "But wait," you say, "didn't a man invent that?" Nineteenth-century American gynecologist J. Marion Sims is often credited with the invention of the speculum, but this is not the case. Sims's speculum looks more like a spoon, while Boivin's speculum, called the *bivalve* for its duckbill design, looks much like the one we use today. It has a self-retaining option so the examiner's hands are free to do a Pap test, which is a very important distinction from Sims's design and somewhat similar to our Roman model. Although she was barred from formally attending medical school in France, her impressive work garnered her an honorary doctorate from the University of Marburg in Germany and led to the early admission of women to medical school in that country. The French, unfortunately, did not recognize her achievements, and she was never admitted into their Académie de Médecine. In fact, her name has essentially been lost to popular history, relegated to university archives and a few websites—at least, that is, until now. *Vive les femmes!*[10]

FIG. 2.6

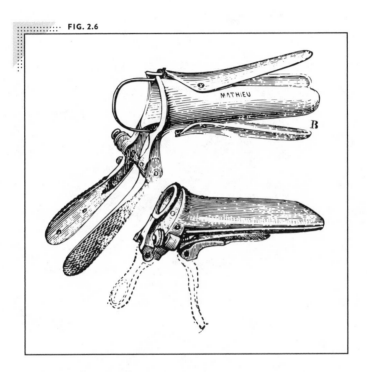

MADAME MARIE BOIVIN'S SPECULUM DESIGN. I ACTUALLY FOUND
THIS EXACT DESIGN STILL IN USE AT MERCY HOSPITAL IN CHICAGO,
AND MOST SELF-RETAINING SPECULA NOW USE A SCREW-DOWN DESIGN.

DID YOU KNOW?

It wasn't until 1994 that the NIH mandated that most clinical trials include women.

3

Bloody Vaginas: A Chapter on Periods

You could see there was blood coming out of her eyes, blood coming out of her. . .wherever.

—THE FORMER 45TH PRESIDENT OF THE
UNITED STATES OF AMERICA

I remember devouring the Judy Blume book, *Are You There God? It's Me, Margaret,* when I was a kid. Blume made periods seem like this amazing rite of passage. What she failed to mention, though, was the pain, the moodiness, and the sheer agony that can occur nearly every month from around age 12 to age 50. We just have to chalk this one up to the way things are, because despite all the advances of modern science, we still menstruate. And after you read this chapter, I hope you will come to understand and embrace your (occasionally) bloody vagina.

WHAT ARE PERIODS, ANYWAY?

As we traverse through life from baby to child to adult, the pituitary gland regulates our growth and entry into puberty. This gland, also nicknamed the master gland, controls and regulates nearly all hormones in the body by releasing cues to tell all the other glands what to do. We are "cycling" all the time—most of the functions our bodies automatically perform daily are results of the pituitary gland producing and regulating hormones involved in many bodily functions, including our sleep cycles. (This amazing gland also has a role in facilitating labor during childbirth.)

Responding to these hormonal cues as we approach puberty, our internal clock tells the pituitary gland to start releasing a certain hormone called GnRH, or gonadotropin-releasing hormone. When this occurs is different for each person and is likely a result of a combination of environment and genetics. The timing has changed over the course of generations as well. The average age for menstruation during the Industrial Revolution (around the 1840s) was 14–17. Today, the average age is 12.5 years, though about 2–3 percent of girls start around age 10.[1]

GnRH is the one hormone that tells the other hormones what to do—release other hormones. More specifically, FSH (follicle-stimulating hormone) stimulates the ovary to release estrogen and the follicles that swell until one releases your egg for that month. In addition, estrogen is responsible for the initial growth of the uterine lining, the endometrium.

After the egg is released from your ovary, what's leftover inside the ovary, called the *corpus luteum*, releases the second major hormone, progesterone. Progesterone is required to help prepare and develop the endometrium, recruiting thousands of tiny blood vessels to encounter a fertilized egg to make sure only the hardiest eggs get to implant and grow. Unfortunately, it's also the hormone that causes the bloating, breast engorgement, and water retention that occurs during the premenstrual phase and pregnancy, as progesterone is what sustains early pregnancy until the placenta is ready to take over providing vital nutritional and hormonal support.

If the egg is not fertilized, which is often the case, hormone levels all drop. Without that hormonal support, the protective uterine lining no longer has a way to sustain itself and therefore simply separates from the host (you). This is menstruation.

········· FIG. 3.1

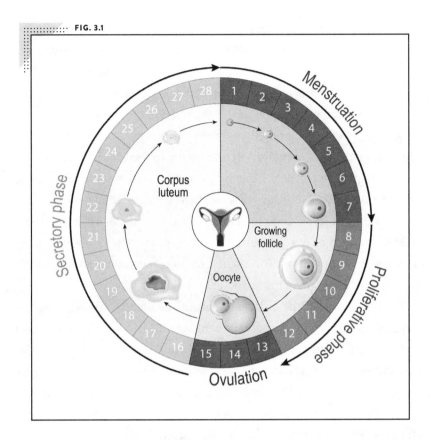

A SCHEMATIC OF THE MENSTRUAL CYCLE, FOLLOWING
AN OOCYTE TO MATURATION

Why do we bleed?

Why must we have bloody vaginas every month in the first place? No one knows absolutely for sure, but there are a couple of good scientific theories that can shed some light on this rather odd and regular occurrence. The main one concerns the phenomenon called *spontaneous decidualization* that occurs once progesterone levels start to go down just before menstruation.

Before you nod off, let's define what this means. The term *decidua* is derived from the Latin verb *decidere*, meaning to die, to fall off, or to detach. Decidualization is simply the process of shedding the uterine lining. In most other mammals, the embryo causes a partial breaking down of the lining in order to implant, and it's easy for an embryo to implant itself. In these mammals, the embryo and developing placenta sit lightly inside the cavity, balancing on the lining, and do not truly access the deep blood vessels of the uterus. By contrast, in humans, the placenta literally invades these deeper layers of the uterus to feed. The theory is that, because humans are genetically more complex, need more nutrients, and are more prone to genetic mistakes, women have evolved methods such as a thicker uterine lining and much more blood and tissue in the uterus per cycle (compared to our primate cousins) to keep some of our unhealthy embryos from implanting. This theory makes certain that if all that energy is getting used, it's going toward actually making a baby.

So it appears that the breaking down of the lining is just a side effect of a genetic adaptation that actually benefits reproduction. Mammals that exhibit spontaneous decidualization share a number of other reproductive characteristics, such as spontaneous ovulation, extended mating (i.e., not going into "heat" like dogs and cats), a placenta that invades maternal blood vessels deeply, and giving birth to only one or two well-developed offspring per pregnancy, as opposed to a litter. This cost/benefit balance (loss of blood from menstruation versus undeveloped or unhealthy offspring) likely explains why this system evolved in only a few species: primarily in humans, some primates, a few bats, and the tiny elephant shrew.[2] Overall, think of your cycles as variations on a central theme: The main event of ovulation happens regularly to allow us greater control over baby making.

Now, sometimes ovulation doesn't happen at all. This occurs when the system is not working as it should. Larger shifts in the delicate balance between estrogen and progesterone can suppress ovulation. Ovulation is the pivotal event in menstruation. If there is no ovulation, the hormones that run the second half of the menstrual cycle don't get made. If those hormones aren't made, then the period or shedding of the uterine lining can't happen on time. During times of stress—and how much stress will affect a cycle varies from person to person—you may not ovulate. This makes sense. If your body isn't primed for such a huge investment of energy such as baby growing, then your body simply shouldn't do it. There are many physiologic reasons why this occurs, but keep this one thought in mind:

No egg = no baby.

One myth I absolutely *must* dispel here is the notion that the body has the ability to get rid of an unwanted pregnancy in certain situations. Several years ago, a certain politician who will not be named here claimed that the body simply "takes care of" pregnancies conceived in rape. Physiology does not work that way. Once you have conceived, pregnancy will generally progress.

IS MY PERIOD IRREGULAR?

Where *did* this mystery idea of 28 days come from? Charles Darwin thought that the 28-day average human menstrual cycle was evidence that our ancestors lived on the seashore and needed to synchronize with the moon and the tides. However, women of reproductive age aren't all walking around bleeding when the moon is full, so this can't possibly be true. What is true is that 28 days is the average lunar month, and the ancients utilized a 13-month calendar of 28-day months each, totaling 364 days a year plus one, which makes 365. The theory for why we menstruate once a month is that there must be some genetic advantage that allows women to exert greater control over when she decides to reproduce.

All this cycling, ovulation, shedding, and so on is a delicate system, and it is by no means perfect. We have been taught to believe that having our menses exactly once a month is normal. After all we've learned, I would like to present an alternate theory. Certainly, periods should come around every month, but to think that any small change in your period or its cycling is somehow indicative of ill health may not be the case.

Certainly, stress can alter your cycles, as well as even minor hormonal changes. Hormones do not operate in a vacuum, and changes happen throughout the month and throughout life. Simply because your hormones may shift somewhat month to month does not mean something is wrong with you. It simply means you're a human woman, imperfect and lovely.

We know that cycles can vary anywhere from 21 to 35 days, and this is all OK. Some women can time their cycles to the moment. For others, their cycles are unpredictable from month to month. This, too, is completely normal.

Lifestyle can affect the timing of your cycle and even your actual flow. There is a study of women in rural southern Poland who generally worked long days during harvest time. It was found that they had lower hormone levels than other women, even though they generally ate the same number of calories, which resulted in fewer and lighter periods. Why is that? Well, if your hormones are somewhat lower, the lining of the uterus is not as thick. If the lining is not thick enough with new blood vessels, it is more difficult for the embryo to implant, since it needs to burrow more deeply. This makes sense because, even though ovulation is still occurring, it's not a good time to grow a baby while you're spending all your energy working. In addition, menstruation can be lighter at this time to lose less energy from blood loss. The body makes its own adjustments without our knowledge. Amazing! Of course, harvest doesn't occur all the time. During other times, the progesterone levels increase, and the lining of the uterus thickens again, signaling that it's OK to implant. These are all theories, but this could explain why some menstrual cycles are heavier or lighter than others.[3]

The most common questions (and complaints) I get from my patients are about minor irregularities in their menstrual cycle. Here is the answer I give the most often. Humans are essentially not that much more evolved than we were a thousand (or even five hundred) years ago. All those years ago, when women were at childbearing age, the majority of them were either pregnant, breastfeeding, or perhaps experiencing some stressor that altered ovulation. During these times, menstruation would be absent. It is my theory that women aren't meant to be menstruating once a month at all—as animals, we should be reproducing, breastfeeding, or perhaps just trying to survive. So it is no surprise to me that periods aren't always exactly 28 days. The normal range is 21–35 days, recognizing that cycles are shifting all the time throughout reproductive life.

IS THERE SOMETHING WRONG WITH ME?

We know that periods aren't perfect and that it's easy and expected to have irregular cycles, so what to do if the periods become *really* hectic? How do we solve this dilemma? When it comes to overly bloody vaginas, there are generally two reasons why this happens: One is a structural problem, meaning some type of excess growth of the endometrial (uterine) lining such as a polyp, and the other is a hormonal imbalance or shift.

Almost every day, I have a patient come to me complaining that she has "estrogen dominance." This misnomer has completely overtaken the internet literature whenever you search for anything related to female hormones, whether in balance or not. The claim is that the most common reason for chronic absence of ovulation, or anovulation (remember, no egg = no baby), is polycystic ovary syndrome (PCOS). Oddly enough, PCOS is not exactly a condition of estrogen dominance but of testosterone (androgen) excess.

How does that work, you ask?

In a normal menstrual cycle, the brain stimulates the ovary to do its thing, which starts as we mentioned before with GnRH, the gonadotropin-releasing hormone. This hormone from the hypothalamus stimulates the pituitary gland to make and release the luteinizing hormone (LH). LH stimulates the ovary to make a pre-testosterone-like hormone that is eventually turned into actual testosterone and then into estrogen.

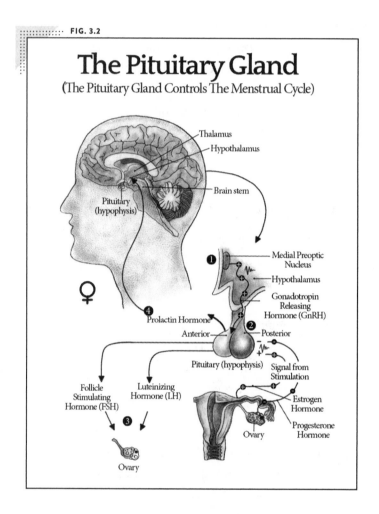

FIG. 3.2

**IN A NUTSHELL, THE BRAIN TELLS THE OVARIES WHAT TO DO,
AND THE OVARIES TELL THE UTERUS WHAT TO DO.**

When things are not working as they should, as in conditions like PCOS, your body makes too much GnRH, which results in too much LH and therefore too much testosterone. Your body doesn't know what else to do with all that extra testosterone, so it turns it into estrogen—which is why the lay media calls this condition estrogen dominance. This is how testosterone is converted into estrogen:

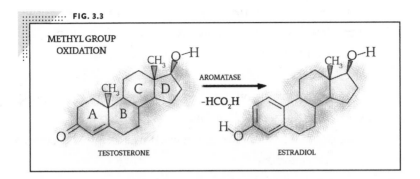

THIS IS HOW YOUR BODY CHANGES TESTOSTERONE TO ESTROGEN (ESTRADIOL).

When there is too much estrogen (estradiol) in the system, the lining of your uterus will continue to grow. Remember, estrogen is responsible for the initial proliferation of the lining. If there is too much estrogen, your body will simply grow more lining for weeks, even months. Another way you get too much estrogen is with the presence of excess adipose (fat). A weaker estrogen called *estrone* comes from fatty tissue and also contributes to the growth of the lining. Therefore, you think you're missing your period while the lining is actually just still growing.

The overgrowth of the uterine lining will eventually outgrow its own blood supply and start to break down, resulting in heavy bleeding, which is perceived as a period. The truth of the matter is, this is not a normal menstrual cycle resulting from a drop in your hormones; the lining keeps growing due to the excess estrogen made from testosterone. As a result, you keep bleeding because estrogen is still stimulating blood and vessel growth until the lining is finally completely spent, which could take weeks or even months. This is the most common cause for the irregularity of cycling when the system is off by abnormal shifts in hormones, such as that of PCOS. If this happens chronically, several other changes can occur: Not only are your periods irregular and heavy, but the excess testosterone can lead to acne, facial and occasionally chest hair growth, and even male pattern hair loss over time.

Issues with ovulation are the most common causes of an irregular, bloody vagina. Now, just because you may skip ovulation occasionally does not mean you have PCOS. However, if it happens on a regular basis, it may be a good idea to see your doc, because the way we diagnose it is not with labs, but with just talking to you. Lab results are helpful, but not actually required. What does this mean? It means that we have done enough study on this particular condition that we can be pretty sure of the diagnosis by observing these three things:

1. Evidence of hyperandrogenism (excess testosterone) such as acne, hair growth, male pattern hair loss, etc.
2. Menstrual irregularities
3. Infertility

There are plenty of other reasons for an irregular period, which include but are not limited to the following:

Pregnancy and breastfeeding

The most common reason for period irregularities is the most physiologic and normal: pregnancy. As we all probably already know, the levels of progesterone in pregnancy skyrocket to support the baby and form the placenta, so that means no periods, in general. Some women do have some irregular spotting at the beginning of a pregnancy, which is most often due to implantation.

Breastfeeding also can cause irregularity in cycles because it suppresses ovulation and menstruation. The theory is that this allows for the body to heal and focus on feeding the current child as opposed to trying to grow another one at the same time.

Just started having periods

If you're new to the bloody vagina game, it can take your body up to an entire year or so to get into some type of pattern. Again, remember, not everyone's cycle is exactly 28 days with 4 days of flow. Just follow your own patterns to see if any particular one bears out.

Weight extremes

Are you obese? Are you too thin? When you are at the extremes of weight, your body has a tough time getting into a pattern. If you are overweight or obese, as we discussed earlier, you have a surplus of hormone that causes the lining to keep growing overtime, which delays the period and makes it longer when it does happen. If you are very thin, with the frame of a ballet dancer, gymnast, or '90s supermodel, your hormone-releasing mechanism is actually suppressed, so there's nothing in the uterus to bleed out. Like in politics, a body likes moderation.

Dietary deficiencies

Do you eat crappy foods and still expect a normal, happy monthly period? While I don't ask my patients this exact question, it is one of the first issues I explore with them when they ask about menstrual irregularities. Garbage in, garbage out. I often tell my patients to eat clean. This is easier (and cheaper) than it sounds. No junk food, no fast food, no soda, I say. It's a great step in the right direction. Here are a few simple rules:

- No food you purchase that comes in a package or in a box that you must reconstitute with water, etc.

- No food from your car window or that a delivery person brings to you in a big, flat box.

- No soda. Ever. Drink water, coconut water, or 100 percent juice of any kind.

By making a few simple changes to your diet, you can improve your health and possibly improve the regularity of your cycle.

MY VAGINA IS TOO BLOODY

If you have an overly bloody vagina with a mostly regular cycle, then we start to think more about the possibility of there being a physical or structural issue with the uterus, vagina, or so on, meaning there is an actual object causing the bleeding, as opposed to some sort of imbalance in your hormones. Some women just bleed a lot, but if you think your vagina is simply *too* bloody, answer the following questions to see if you need to visit your doctor:

1. Do you find yourself changing your pad/tampon/cup every hour or two?
2. Do you get up in the middle of the night with stained sheets during your period?
3. Do you use double protection (meaning two pads, tampon and pad, cup and pad, etc.)?
4. Is your period longer than seven days?
5. Do you limit social activities because you are afraid you may leak through your pad/tampon/cup?
6. Do you feel tired or listless or have a lack of energy during your period?
7. Have you ever missed work or school because of your period?

If you answer yes to many of these questions, then your vagina might be a bit too bloody, and it's time to see your doc and find out what's the matter. In order to explore this in more detail, let's break down the possibilities so it makes more sense. Physical conditions that can cause a bloody vagina include the following:

Polyp

Polyps are little benign growths and are basically the same as colon or nasal polyps. Sometimes they go away with a heavy period or they may need to be removed if they persist.

Adenomyosis

Adenomyosis causes painful and very bloody vaginas. It occurs when the blood vessels and tissue that usually come out each month start to invade the uterus. This makes the organ larger and mushier and less like the muscle that it is, so when it's time for a period, the uterus must contract even more strongly because it cannot work like it's supposed to. Since the uterus can't contract down to become small again, there's more bleeding every month.

Fibroids

Fibroids are incredibly common. You probably know someone with fibroids or have one or two yourself (if you have a uterus). I do. They happen in about 30 percent of White women and up to 50 percent of women of African descent, mostly beginning in their mid-twenties, and they can cause a seriously bloody vagina. Usually benign muscle growths, when small they are virtually undetectable and cause no symptoms, but over time, they can grow to be larger than grapefruits.

Cancer

Cancer. Ugh. We suspect cancer if there is persistent bleeding in a woman with risk factors such as chronic androgen/estrogen imbalance or bleeding in any woman who has made it into menopause. Pain. Weight loss. Fatigue—see a doctor. But the good news is, if caught early, survival can exceed 90 percent.

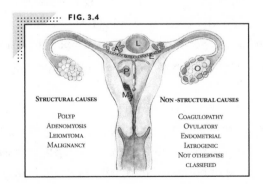

FIG. 3.4

STRUCTURAL CAUSES

POLYP
ADENOMYOSIS
LEIOMYOMA
MALIGNANCY

NON-STRUCTURAL CAUSES

COAGULOPATHY
OVULATORY
ENDOMETRIAL
IATROGENIC
NOT OTHERWISE
CLASSIFIED

ILLUSTRATION OF THE VARIOUS CAUSES OF A BLOODY VAGINA.

Non-physical causes for a too-bloody vagina include the following:

Coagulopathy

A coagulopathy is a disorder in a person's ability to clot blood. No, this does not refer to the blood clots that may come out during a menstrual cycle, but rather to the body's ability to stop tiny blood vessels from bleeding by forming a clot. In some conditions, such as von Willebrand disease, you can't easily stop bleeding, which could result in long, heavy menstrual cycles. Once discovered, there are many ways to treat conditions such as these.

Ovulatory

The most common ovulatory reason for heavy cycles is anovulation. Remember, if you do not release your egg for the month, the body doesn't know to proceed to the second half of the menstrual cycle, so the lining keeps growing. This results in long, heavy periods of bleeding. Treatments for ovulatory problems may vary, but most often include finding a way to either promote ovulation or to mimic it with medication, lifestyle changes such as weight control, or both.

Endometrial

In an otherwise normal-cycling woman who has been shown to be ovulating, one may encounter bleeding or spotting in between periods, or simply heavy menstrual bleeding. We then consider the possibility that there's some problem with the way the endometrium itself develops. If you have spotting at ovulation, this could be coming from a small drop in estrogen at ovulation and is not a disorder, but we don't want to dismiss it and we include it in this classification when counseling our patients.

Iatrogenic

The term *iatrogenic* means something that a medical treatment caused. You can get irregular periods from a hormone-containing IUD, or even when you start taking any type of hormonal birth control. Periods may also become heavier if you choose to use a copper-containing IUD. While most of the hormonal causes of irregular periods improve over time, these causes can be rectified by changing or discontinuing the treatment in question.

Not otherwise classified

Modern medicine always includes a catch-all, just in case we forget something or have yet to discover something new. That's where "not otherwise classified" comes in.

THE SISTERHOOD CYCLING THEORY

One interesting theory about periods that is still around today is the sisterhood cycling theory, which proposes that women's periods synchronize when living together. In 1971, an article by Dr. Martha McClintock detailing these findings was published in the journal *Nature*.[4] This article has been cited thousands of times, but it remains controversial and largely unproven, despite its assimilation into popular culture. The most prominent theory was that it was an evolutionary strategy among females to cooperate with each other. If women were all cycling together, it was unlikely that one man could reproduce with them all in one go, therefore protecting them against becoming part of a harem. Given that the early 1970s saw the burgeoning women's rights movement, this theory of period sisterhood gained a lot of popularity.

The study took a bunch of women in a college dormitory and followed them over several months. Of the sample of 312 women, 244 had cycles that were longer than 29 days or shorter than 27, and only 70 percent of the rest actually started their period within two weeks of the full moon. Since not everyone's cycles are 28 days long, as we previously explained, it did appear like there was some type of social period cooperation, as periods will naturally overlap given enough time.[5]

Some academics recently decided to find out if the findings of synchronicity of periods could be put down to chance or if it's a real phenomenon.

One study looked at six years' worth of data on the menstrual cycles of our close cousins, baboons.

Two models were proposed: The first one was the period sisterhood hypothesis (defense against becoming part of a harem) and the other was the boring hypothesis, which asserts that the phenomenon could occur by chance. By doing lots of math, the researchers compared how much each model would account for the data they discovered. They found that the model assuming that patterns would appear by chance was statistically the best model. Think about it—if you have a large number of women with varying cycle lengths and only approximately 21–35 days in a lunar month, of course many women will be menstruating together at some point in time. It appears that chance is the winner here.[6]

Unfortunately, we were still talking about this in the literature as late as 2005, and any search on "cycling together" will reveal and promote this theory.[7]

There was an alternate theory proposed by Dr. Chris Knight: Menstruation did, once upon a time, synchronize in early cultures, but we evolved away from it over time as we moved from hunting to farming. How is this explained? In early cultures, we were hunter-gatherers, and the ability to obtain meat and therefore increase fitness and survival of the species was paramount. The theory goes that in order for females to obtain enough meat to feed themselves and their unborn children, they needed to exercise their sexual power over men, the hunters, by withholding sex en masse at menstruation. The men needed to bring the meat back to demonstrate their fitness for procreation. This is an interesting theory, but of course completely unprovable.[8]

MYTHS ABOUT BLOODY VAGINAS

Despite how common menstruation is and the generations of women who have had them, myths, social stigma, and shame abound, both in the US and abroad. These taboos appear from the earliest writings and teachings across the ages. As we will see, there is a range of thought. For example, take this Bible excerpt from Leviticus 15:

[19] When a woman has her regular flow of blood, the impurity of her monthly period will last seven days, and anyone who touches her will be unclean till evening. [20] Anything she lies on during her period will be unclean, and anything she sits on will be unclean. [21] Anyone who touches her bed will be unclean; they must wash their clothes and bathe with water, and they will be unclean till evening. [22] Anyone who touches anything she sits on will be unclean; they must wash their clothes and bathe with water, and they will be unclean till evening. [23] Whether it is the bed or anything she was sitting on, when anyone touches it, they will be unclean till evening. [24] If a man has sexual relations with her and her monthly flow touches him, he will be unclean for seven days; any bed he lies on will be unclean.

Or how about this from the Quran 2:222:

They ask you about menstruation. Say: It is a state of impurity; so keep away from women in the state of menstruation, [238] and do not approach them until they are cleansed. And when they are cleansed, [239] then come to them as Allah has commanded you. [240] Truly, Allah loves those who abstain from evil and keep themselves pure.

According to the Mishnah, a component of the Talmud, a Jewish text, there are thirty-six transgressions that may possibly be punished by death. Number one is sex with one's mother. Number fifteen is sex with a woman while she is menstruating.

Ancient Rome is not to be left out. Pliny the Elder was an "expert" on natural history during those times, and he also believed menstrual fluid to be a little more than problematic:

> *Contact with it turns new wine sour, crops touched by it become barren, grafts die, seed in gardens are dried up, the fruit of trees falls off, the edge of steel and the gleam of ivory are dulled, hives of bees die, even bronze and iron are at once seized by rust, and a horrible smell fills the air; to taste it drives dogs mad and infects their bites with an incurable poison.*
> —*From* Natural History: A Selection, *by Pliny the Elder*

If this were really the case—because at any given time on earth there is a menstruating woman—then nothing would ever grow and we would have all already starved to death.

According to some 5th/4th century BCE Hippocratic texts, women's flesh is more like a sponge than men's flesh, so it actually can absorb more fluid from what is eaten and drunk, and then that fluid builds up all month, and what goes in must come out. The belief is if it doesn't come out, women will become ill, as the blood could rot or migrate somewhere in the body—just like that wandering uterus—and put pressure on vital organs.[9]

Although we have evolved somewhat from ancient and biblical times, period shaming and myth have persisted through the centuries. For example, in Vienna during the 1920s, there was a doctor by the name of Schick (he is most famous for the "Schick test" used to detect immunity to diphtheria toxin). According to lore, one day a patient sent him flowers as a thank you. When the good doctor asked his nurse to put them in water, she told him she couldn't because she was menstruating, and she didn't want them to wilt. Whether or not she believed this or was being sarcastic to avoid doing non-nursing work, or even if this is the real version of the story, we will never know. Regardless, this caused Dr. Schick to land upon the theory known as *menotoxin*. This ridiculous theory supposes that women having their periods excrete something that literally kills things.

Here's how the experiment allegedly worked. Dr. Schick gave subjects each three flowers. Within a few minutes, those flowers began to wilt, and within a day, they had died. Of course, flowers will die if they're not put in water, regardless of who is holding them.

A similar experiment showed that menstruating women's dough for bread-making did not rise as high as that of non-menstruating women. Again, no control for outside factors were taken into account. These flawed experiments are true examples of how a researcher can make their outcomes work however they want depending on their own beliefs. All we get is a self-fulfilling prophecy. The doctor wanted to prove women were toxic during menstruation, so he did. Of course, we came to our senses later in the century, right? Actually, no. *The Lancet*, a respected British journal featured a written debate about menstrual pollution (AKA menotoxin) as late as 1974. One (female) doctor, Virginia Ernster, wrote in and finally put this particular discussion to rest: "A 1924 photograph of a wilted daisy . . . and the unexplainable death of one Italian tree . . . are insufficient data on which to build a case in 1974."[12]

Or so we thought. In 2005, a sign was posted at a swimming pool in Georgia (the country, not the state) strongly recommending that women refrain from swimming. It stated: "Dear Ladies! Do not go to the pool during periods."[13] And during the 2016 Olympics, when swimmer Fu Yuanhui from China admitted she was having her period during the competition, the Chinese internet went mad with comments. Many were expressing surprise that women were even allowed to swim during their period without spoiling the water. Some even questioned why the pool didn't turn red.[14]

Thus the myth of menotoxin persists to this day. Of course, the fitness center said that it was to protect their customers due to a "contamination" of menstrual blood in the pool. More likely than not, swimming pool issues come from a lack of proper cleaning and chlorination. Bacteria from other sources, often from fecal matter or urine, which everyone makes, can proliferate in standing water that is not properly cleaned, NOT from a vagina simply doing what it does. In fact, menstrual blood has no odor until after it has come in contact with air.

Again, to reiterate—here are activities you can't do when you have a bloody vagina: **Nothing.**

Now, not all bloody vagina myths are negative. In some cultures, there are positive associations with menstruation, which is something I want to begin to perpetuate once more in the here and now. In certain cultures, the ability to bleed for several days without dying demonstrates fertility and power, and menstruation has magical properties.

In Aboriginal Australian culture and some other traditional cultures, men, in the course of initiation rites, must learn to "menstruate" symbolically as their basic means of asserting ritual potency. There is also a theory that circumcision arose from the thinking that men's release of blood gave them power and fertility like that of a female.[15]

The secrets of wisdom and divinity are associated with menstruation in many other ancient cultures the world over. Some ancient West African traditions say that menstrual blood is "congealed to form a man," denoting the power of creation that results from a woman's ability to menstruate. In fact, even today among the Ashanti tribe in West Africa, girls are held in high regard because they are the carriers of *mogya*, the blood.

The Norse god Thor achieved enlightenment and immortality by bathing in the menstrual blood of the "giantess."

Indigenous peoples of South America said that all mankind was made of "moon blood" in the beginning.

The Chinese philosophy of Taoism taught that a man could become immortal by drinking or absorbing menstrual blood, called red yin juice, from a woman's "mysterious gateway." Ancient Taoists also considered red a sacred color, which persists to this day. Traditional Chinese (and Indian) wedding ceremonies usually feature a bride decked out in red. Perhaps the modern Chinese internet users should look back at their own culture for positive period associations.

It is possible that the rituals of drinking or bathing in blood are where the idea of bloodletting to treat disease originated. It is known that with the onset of menstruation, bleeding relieves some of the symptoms of PMS. Practitioners may have extrapolated that inducing bleeding can help everything. The concept of bloodletting originated more than three thousand years ago and allegedly came from a need to balance the "humours" in the body. In this way, it may have its origins in women's bloody vaginas, as your "humours" may not be as "humorous" once the period begins. So using a leech to aid in the bleeding process now seems to make sense as a way to achieve the desired result more quickly.

DO HOME REMEDIES ACTUALLY WORK?

Since we're out to dispel myths about bloody vaginas, let us review a short list of the things that I've heard my patients use for their various bloody vagina issues and whether or not they're any good.

- Blackstrap molasses: Doesn't slow the flow as some believe, but contains iron that helps to support the blood loss and tastes sweet.
- Probiotics: Can help with constipation and maybe some other GI issues associated with pre-menstruation.
- Becoming vegetarian or following the Mediterranean diet: Could be a healthy lifestyle choice, and the Omega-3s are always useful in supporting overall health. There are some small studies that show Omega-3s may help somewhat with painful cycles.
- DIM supplement: Has not been studied and needs more information; theoretically helpful though.
- Avoiding milk and dairy: Makes sense only if you're lactose intolerant. Consider modification if you're really gassy after indulging in that Brie. There hasn't been a single study to support stopping dairy products. Milk does a body good!
- Adding milk and dairy: Yes, that may seem odd, given that dairy

has such a bad name associated with period problems, but a study showed that painful periods and other symptoms were found in significantly fewer female students who consumed three or four servings of dairy products per day as compared to participants who consumed no dairy products.

- Weight loss: Always useful if you're overweight and can help decrease androgens like testosterone, which is turned into estrogen. This extra estrogen can throw off the delicate hormone balance. If weight is reduced, it may therefore reduce menstrual irregularity.
- Castor oil: Made for constipation and tastes disgusting. Take it only if you really need to go.
- Traditional Chinese Medicine: There are varying formulas and instructions for taking these preparations depending upon the practitioner, making it difficult to standardize across a population and study en masse. I have seen varying degrees of success from my patients' self-reporting.
- Green tea: Is delicious, so it can't hurt, and may have some anti-inflammatory properties.
- Vitamin supplements such as E, C, B complex, and D: Can't hurt unless you take massive amounts. There are a few supportive studies on these. Just take a multivitamin every day.
- Flax and sesame seeds: Although more associated with anticancer properties, they have been shown to decrease sex hormones like testosterone and may help treat conditions like PCOS. There isn't a single shred of evidence that "seed cycling" makes your period any less bloody, though.

With all of this information in mind, in actuality, few home remedies have been proven to help decrease the flow of a bloody vagina. Most of these have more to do with increasing your overall health than actually stopping bleeding. Since on the whole there is little harm with trying these, and since the placebo effect is often strong, and as long as someone is monitoring your progress, you'll probably be OK if you want to try them. However, exercise common sense. For example, if you have diabetes, don't take the sweet blackstrap molasses.

You should also consider that going through lists like this can make life even more complicated than it already is, and I want you to be able to be healthy with a regular period without having to consult a book. So my advice is simply this: Eat clean, use extra virgin olive oil for cooking (more on this below), and take a multivitamin.[16] If the food you intend to eat comes from a box or some other long-term storage mechanism, or it comes in one form and you have to add water to reconstitute it, or you can't pronounce the ingredients, avoid it.[17]

SOME REMEDIES THAT DO WORK

Now, there are a few over-the-counter remedies that we have actual data for, and I'm more than happy to offer you a couple of options here:

- Ibuprofen (or any NSAID): Ibuprofen taken several hours before or the day your period begins has been proven to help decrease flow by up to 30 percent. The mechanism is probably due to the anti-inflammatory properties of NSAIDs. It's the most popular way to handle cramps for a pretty good reason—it works!
- Chasteberry (also known by its scientific name, Vitex): This has some supportive studies that it helps with period symptoms such as bloating, mood swings, and breast tenderness when taken about two weeks before the flow.
- Get some exercise: Specifically aerobic or cardio exercise has been proven to help with painful bloody vaginas because pain mediators decrease with an increase in exercise. Progesterone, the balancer to estrogen, also increases with exercise. However you get your heart pumping—spinning, running, whatever you enjoy—will be helpful for those annoying symptoms.

- Warm her up: Break out that old heating pad, it really helps. Also, a good hot bath with your relaxing scent of choice and a bit of baking soda can also offer relief if you don't have a heating pad. Add a little clary sage oil for a calming effect.

- Vitamins: Simply take a multivitamin. There are a few individual supplements such as zinc, magnesium, vitamin D, vitamin E, and fish oil that do have some supportive studies on crampy pain during the bloody vagina time. Magnesium may help to decrease the detection of pain, and zinc seems to reduce cramps. But taking individual supplements can be difficult and expensive over time. Get a daily women's multivitamin from the drugstore and take it every day.

- Olive oil: There have been some supportive studies showing that eating about 25cc's (about 5 teaspoons) of extra virgin olive oil a day helps to decrease painful menstrual cramps, otherwise known as primary dysmenorrhea. While the studies did not look at the heaviness of cycles, I find this information helpful as less cramping often leads to less bleeding.

HOW TO CARE FOR MY BLOODY VAGINA

It never ceases to amaze me how much misinformation exists about the "best" way to care for yourself during menstruation. From those truly weird videos in the 1960s and 1970s telling us "you're becoming a woman now" to internet ads on how to "feel fresh," myths about menstrual care are seemingly endless.

According to a 2015 CDC study, 62 percent of American women surveyed use pads, compared with 42 percent who use tampons.[18] This statistic actually shocked me. I find tampons to be the most convenient menstrual product, so why more modern American women choose pads for their bloody vagina management eludes me, but I have a few theories as to why. Perhaps it's to track the flow better? Maybe they are scared they will get toxic shock syndrome? Maybe it's feeling uncomfortable with their own anatomy. If that is the case, I hope this book can help in some small way. Regardless of your choice, at least we have choices.

Menstrual pads have evolved over the years from being bulky and diaper-like to being ultra-thin, barely detectable marvels. Now, these ultra-thin pads would not be possible without science, and that means they use plastic and synthetics. That top layer that keeps you super dry? That's synthetic. That absorbent core? It may look like cotton, but that's synthetic too, often blended with rayon, a derivative of cellulose. Cellulose is the most common organic compound on earth. While usually used to make paper, cellulose also has absorbent properties, which makes it ideal for pads. Now what's the stuff at the bottom? That's plastic. All that being said, it's a bit of a necessity in our bloody vagina world, and given their increased absorbency we now are using somewhat fewer pads per cycle, which is a good thing for the environment. Use of synthetics also keeps costs down, and with the tampon tax (more on that soon), we need it! Of course, we have other options, and in recent years, women are beginning to turn to other products such as organic tampons, menstrual cups, period underwear, and reusables.

Organic pads

These pads usually contain a combination of cotton and cellulose. Although there is no data to indicate that these types of pads are less irritating, if you have found through your experience with other pads that you are sensitive, it may be worth a go. Not to mention there is a "feel good" mentality to them that is certainly appealing, and the fact that they are made from smaller companies helps to support innovation. These smaller companies do come with a cost, and since organic cotton is more labor intensive to produce, these pads are more expensive. Given this knowledge, the choice is up to you.

Reusable pads

Reusable pads may be a good option, especially for women in low-re-source countries or those who are housing insecure. Companies such as

Lunapads, Afripads, and Gladrags are pioneering this movement. Additionally, these reusable products are good for the environment and pollute less, especially because they lack the plastic backing.

Tampons

Tampons are my personal favorite. The earliest documented use of intravaginal menstrual care, the tampon, dates back to ancient Egypt where women used rolled papyrus wrapped around a small twig. Romans used rolled wool tucked inside. The modern tampon as we know it was invented in 1929 by Dr. Earle Haas and was originally made of cotton and wool. While the material composition was not much different from the tampons the Romans used, at least he attached a string, to avoid the dreaded lost tampon. They have since evolved to be made primarily of a rayon/cotton composite, a much more absorbent material. You might have heard that rayon can contain a cancer-causing chemical called dioxin. Rayon is now made using a chlorine-limiting or chlorine-free process monitored by the FDA to limit dioxin production, and in fact, even all 100 percent cotton can have trace amounts of dioxin. The FDA website reports that the dioxin in the rayon raw materials ranges from an undetectable 0.1 to 1 part per trillion, which is incredibly tiny. So know that these trace amounts in your tampons are very unlikely to cause cancer, especially when such amounts of dioxin can also easily be found in the air, water, and ground from past pollutants.[19]

Some makers of organic tampons claim their natural fibers decrease the risk of toxic shock syndrome (TSS), a condition that caused the death of some women in the early 1980s. However, this was linked to a very specific brand of tampon made with a synthetic material (Rely by Proctor and Gamble) and since they were pulled from the shelves, toxic shock has been incredibly rare, in the realm of 1 in 100,000 menstruating women. TSS got a lot of attention around 1979, when 1,300 women were diagnosed with this sometimes fatal condition. Unfortunately, it took the FDA a few years to finally get involved to regulate and test tampon companies more appropriately. This has resulted in the "regular," "super," and "super plus" designations that we know and may grumble about today.[20]

So, while organic tampon makers like to claim that the organic material somehow lowers your risk of toxic shock syndrome, we now know that is not necessarily the case. When researchers actually looked at eleven different types of (modern, post-1980s) tampons and even four types of menstrual cups, they discovered that organic, cotton, rayon, or any blend doesn't make a bit of difference when it comes to the growth of the dangerous bacteria *Staphylococcus aureus* that causes toxic shock syndrome.[21]

Menstrual cups

If you're looking for environmentally friendly, this may be your best option. Menstrual cups are made from medical-grade silicone and may be washed and reused. I use plain dishwashing detergent and hot water for mine. They're also a cost-friendly option at around thirty dollars each, and they last many years. If you can get over the glob of blood you have to pour into the toilet, making changing it a likely at-home activity, it can really save over the long term.

Period underwear

Interestingly, one of the original inventors of period panties, which are supposed to take the place of pads, was a chemical engineering student. What a way to make use of your degree. From my research, period panties appear to be made of multiple layers of fabric, which work to pull menstrual fluid away from your skin and hold it there. These layers are made of a microfiber polyester that traps liquid, which then has to navigate through a maze of tiny filaments as it moves through the material, so it goes really slowly, keeping it from making it to the other side and leaking. The product ads say they can hold up to three teaspoons of liquid at a time. I believe it's a great idea, but like the menstrual cup, the starting price (around thirty dollars) and its lack of availability in undeveloped countries so far makes period underwear a first-world luxury.[22] Perhaps for the unhoused, however, period underwear may be far more attractive and useful than a cup. We must always remember that there are those around us who don't even have the luxury of being able to buy tampons and pads.

THE TAMPON TAX

Bloody vaginas are big business and generate enormous amounts of tax revenue for states that continue to levy taxes on women's menstrual products—as "luxury items," no less. American women spend over $2 billion on menstrual products a year. Over the course of our lives, women will use about seventeen thousand pads and tampons and personally spend more than two thousand dollars on these products.

In many states, sanitary products are not covered by food stamps. For women experiencing housing insecurity or living below the poverty line, the tampon tax may mean choosing between food and pads. Imprisoned women in some states in the US are only allowed a certain number of pads per month and must find other ways to manage the flow or end up free bleeding. This puts low-income and housing-insecure women at particular risk. Because of this tax, women in those states can expect to spend an additional $150 million on something that is essentially a necessity.

As of this printing, here are the states that tax menstrual products. The tide is beginning to turn, but if you live in one of these states that still tax your bloody vagina, let them know how you feel about it.

Alabama	Kansas	North Dakota
Arizona	Kentucky	Oklahoma
Arkansas	Louisiana	South Carolina
Colorado (except the city of Denver)	Maine	Tennessee
Georgia	Michigan	Texas
Hawaii	Mississippi	Vermont
Idaho	Missouri	Virginia
Indiana	Nebraska	Washington
Indiana	New Mexico	West Virginia
Iowa	North Carolina	Wisconsin

MENSTRUAL SEQUESTRATION

Unfortunately, period misconceptions and myths continue to plague women not only in the US but around the world, and safe products are often unavailable. In modern-day India, eight out of ten women and girls live in communities where they are not allowed into a religious shrine while menstruating. Six out of ten are not allowed to touch food in the kitchen, and three out of ten women and girls in modern-day India must sleep in a separate room. This practice of separation goes even further in some other countries.[23]

In some remote villages in countries such as Nepal, the age-old practice of *chhaupadi* (pronounced CHOW-pa-dee), or menstrual sequestration, is still practiced. The word is derived from Nepalese and means someone who bears an impurity. This practice forces menstruating women to separate themselves from their families during menstruation. No one is allowed to even touch them.

These practices are demeaning, and they aid in enshrining a patriarchal hierarchy that means women will always remain second-class citizens in these cultures. Several women have even died of exposure from spending their days in small, poorly ventilated and insulated *chhaupadi* huts. Having no heat source, a 16-year-old-girl died from smoke inhalation after starting a fire to keep warm during a particularly frigid night in her hut. As a result of this tragedy and global pressures, the practice is officially banned, but it will take many years for communities to unlearn these practices.[24]

As people who bleed for several days a month and still manage not to die, it is incumbent upon us all to be open, honest, and forthcoming about our bloody vaginas. Letting people who don't own bloody vaginas make us feel like second-class citizens will only widen the chasm and keep us from achieving all we are capable of. Understanding these natural processes, working with them, and even controlling them when necessary is our right as vagina owners.[25]

Bloody Vagina FAQs

- **I just started my period, and it's irregular. Is this normal?** Yes! It can take up to three to five years after menstruation begins to fall into some type of regularity, which may be anywhere between 21–35 days and can vary a little from month to month. Expect some irregularity with changes in lifestyle, stress, weight, or even diet.

- **Is my cycle too heavy? How can you tell how much is too much?** The average menstrual cycle results in about 80 milliliters of blood and tissue per period. To quantify, 80 milliliters is about 2.7 fluid ounces or about a third of a cup. If you get dizzy, short of breath, or fatigued with menstruation, or if you change products every hour or so, then yes, you may be bleeding too much and seeing a doctor is your best bet to discuss what can be done.[26]

- **My period stinks, and I think I have an infection!** Tissue breaks down; and of course it's going to stink if left to air over time. Interestingly, only about 30 percent of the stuff that comes out during any cycle is actually blood. The rest is tissue, and just like any other tissue that breaks down, once separated from its blood supply and left to sit in a warm environment for some time, odor may result. Think about changing protection more often or switching to a cup or tampon if this continues to be the case. It's very difficult to tell the difference between an infection and flow by just looking, so don't jump the gun.

- **I've never had penetrative sex. Can I use a tampon or menstrual cup?** The hymen, which we discussed earlier, is just vestigial physiology, a part of the body that we do not need, like an appendix. Whether or not it is broken means nothing when it comes to making your bloody vagina as comfortable as possible. So if the mood strikes, stick one in.

- **Can I perm or relax my hair when I'm on my period?** Yes. Your perm or relaxer will take.

- **Do I need to douche after my period?** No! Douching can kill the healthy bacteria, *Lactobacilli*, in your vagina, which can lead to infection. Cleaning the outside of the vagina regularly with a mild soap is OK, but not multiple times a day, as you can strip this very sensitive area of natural oils and end up with an itchy vagina.

DID YOU KNOW?

A 2018 survey revealed that 42 percent of US women say they have experienced period-shaming by men.[27]

4

Vagina Care
(and the Hair Down There)

What do you recommend for detoxifying my vagina?

—THEM

Your vagina isn't toxic.

—ME

The modern information age has brought us many things. With a few keystrokes you can find seemingly endless knowledge on endless subjects, and what people think is good for your vagina is no exception. Unfortunately, included with this information is a bevy of misinformation. The internet and its many product placements have been artfully crafted to relieve you of your money, promising an utterly "detoxified" and pristine and perfect vagina. I want to be as clear as possible about what your vagina needs, and what she does *not*, because most of the time, she needs very little. (And remember, just say no to baby wipes!)

DESTROY GERMS AND ODORS . . . PLEASE

Unfortunately, companies trying to sell women products claiming to remove smells and stop discharge coming from their vaginas are nothing new. This has gone on for many years and includes products such as douches, panty liners, and, at one time, Lysol. Did you know that Lysol was originally marketed as a vaginal disinfectant? In the 1920s, Lysol was advertised as a women's hygiene product to destroy germs and odors. What they are probably insinuating is that women's vaginas are the cause of an unhappy marriage because of the wife's unruly, smelly vagina, and she needs to use Lysol to create a happy home. Unfortunately, when taken in the higher concentrations that this particular disinfectant would likely have had been back then (they have since changed the formula), it can cause severe burning and irritation, killing basically everything in there, sperm included. Lysol was also used after sex for "disinfecting" a vagina full of sperm that could result in an unwanted pregnancy. It didn't work that well, however, making this a don't-try-this-at-home moment.

Lysol was also used in the 1930s to keep a clean vagina after birth. In his 1938 textbook, American obstetric physician Dr. Joseph Bolivar DeLee encouraged the use of Lysol during labor: "[J]ust before introducing the hand, the vagina is liberally flushed with 1 percent lysol solution squeezed from pledgets of cotton, the idea being to reduce the amount of infectious matter unavoidably carried into the puerperal wounds and up into the uterus by the manipulations."[1]

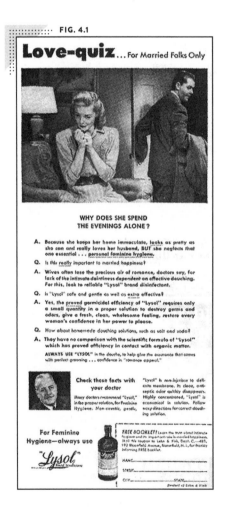

FIG. 4.1

LYSOL DOUCHE NEWSPAPER AD, CIRCA 1948

Thank goodness we invented better things for that, like antibiotics—and gloves.

BUT WHAT IF I DON'T FEEL SO FRESH?

My patients often ask me about how to care for a vagina that doesn't quite feel "fresh." In my humble opinion, I believe that the concept of freshness is preposterous. We have been taught that unless our vaginas smell like open fields of daisies or powder or shower gel, then we are diseased or unhealthy. This harkens right back to the Lysol ad and has been propagated ever since.

Of course, women are nothing more than consumers to the companies that try to sell them these products. And the women who buy more are worth more to them. Therefore, this fear of not being "fresh" is used to this very day to scare women into believing that a panty liner must be worn *daily* to keep the "freshness" going. There has never been any study to prove that wearing a panty liner every day will somehow keep your pH balanced or make your vagina "fresh." I was just doing a quick search on daily panty liner use. What pops up? A well-known product from a trusted brand urges you to "feel shower fresh every day." Here's another kicker from their website, advertising a panty liner for a thong that reads something like this: "For long-lasting freshness whether you're at work or at play, try _____ Thong Daily Liners for discreet protection against daily discharge and odors."

What? It's no wonder my office is jam-packed with women who have so many questions, having been bombarded with ads since before puberty about their malicious "odors" and hideous "discharge." No one needs a daily panty liner. These companies just want you to think you do. Think about this: If you wear a panty liner every day, the average cost is about 15 cents a day. Multiply that by 365, and that's $54.75 a year for a single woman. Now that may not be much to you, but what if all women in the US who do this suddenly stopped buying them? Since I do not have the sales numbers from this company, I can only go on what I see in my office. About 10 percent of my patients wear a daily panty liner; multiplied across the female population of the US, that's 15 million women. If these women understood that it's the liner that is probably causing more issues, hopefully they would stop using them. As a result, if all 15 million women stopped buying daily liners, we have not only just deprived a corporation of more than $800 million dollars earned from misinformation, but we have also saved an entire landfill while freeing vaginas across the nation.

THE BASICS: SOAP, WATER, AND SUNSHINE

I understand how important it is to take charge of your vaginal health, and I am here to help you do just that without spending the literally billions of dollars that women in the US spend on things to somehow improve an already healthy vagina. Vaginal health comes from regular health. When you are well hydrated and oxygenated, so is your vagina. And no, she doesn't always smell like daisies. Consider her a self-cleaning oven. No yoni eggs, pearls, or anything similar to detoxify your already wonderful vagina are required.

What your vagina really needs to flourish is actually pretty basic. First, she needs water—and no, not for douching. We will cover douching in more depth in chapter 6, when we discuss yeast infections, but please know for now that you shouldn't be douching, ever.

Many of my patients come into the office complaining of vaginal discharge. And while most discharge is actually normal—simple reactions to hormonal shifts, diet, clothing choices, and so on—the most common cause of a change in your discharge that I have found is dehydration. The water you take in serves to feed your cells and keep them working properly. When deprived of water, the cells in your vagina are unable to make enough fluid to keep you well lubricated and healthy with a balanced pH. In addition, that water helps your healthy vaginal bacteria, *Lactobacilli*. The discharge that is made when you're dehydrated is much thicker and more viscous and may have a different smell, primarily because it's so concentrated. A good rule of thumb is this: After you urinate, check the toilet. Your urine should be pale yellow. If it's darker than that, drink more water. Your vagina (and your many other organs) will thank you.

Water is also an important part of external vaginal, or vulvar, cleaning. But what should you use as a cleaning product when washing down there? There are literally hundreds of products that have been marketed to make you think your vagina is a bad place, an unruly, unclean, bacteria-ridden place that must be conquered. Of course, she is bacteria laden, but not all bacteria are bad. Your vagina is just fine, and she will treat you fine as long as you treat her right. There's absolutely no need for you to use anything other than warm (not hot) water and basic soap. Yes, you read that right, just soap. And the best kind of soap to use is one with as few ingredients as possible, such as a bar soap like Dove, Ivory, or something similar. Your vagina is simply skin. She has special skin, but it is just skin, and it needs normal, routine cleaning. Use a soft washcloth or just your hand—no shower scrubbers as you could irritate the skin and cause itching. Dry her well by patting, and don't forget a mild moisturizer, preferably unscented, especially if you shave.

The one other thing I recommend as a necessity for vagina care is letting the sunshine in. This means making sure to let her get plenty of air. Stifling your vagina with layers of non-breathable clothing such as leggings, jeggings, tights, and thong underwear is a one-way ticket to irritation and the gyno's office. When you come home from work, gym, or barre class, peel off those clingy clothes and give her a little sun. At night, leave the underwear off and give her a little moonshine too. As for thongs . . . well, only wear them when you plan on taking them off shortly.

That's right—that's it. The three main things your vagina needs are soap, water, and sunshine, much like the rest of your skin. Certainly, depending on the vagina, there may be some additions or changes that need to be made, but overall, your very special vagina needs some very basic things and should be treated as part of you, not some otherworldly, special area that somehow needs expensive products to make and keep her happy.

And I must mention here, with regard to putting things inside your vagina, think of this rule of thumb: If you can eat it, don't put it in there. If you can smoke it, don't put it in there. If you can drink it, well, you get the idea.

SHOULD I SHAVE DOWN THERE?

I would be remiss if I didn't also discuss pubic hair and hair removal. The human body contains 5 million hair follicles, composed of two types, vellus hair and terminal hair. Vellus hairs are the very fine hairs that cover basically everything and are barely perceptible. Terminal hairs are darker and more noticeable. Terminal hairs develop at puberty in the armpit and pubic area with the addition of testosterone (androgens). Terminal hairs are also associated with glands and nerve endings.

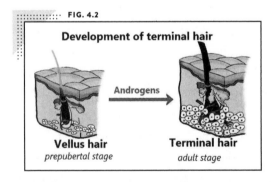

FIG. 4.2

Development of terminal hair

Androgens

Vellus hair
prepubertal stage

Terminal hair
adult stage

AFTER THE ADDITION OF ANDROGEN (TESTOSTERONE),
HAIR BECOMES THICKER AND DARKER.

This hair is actually there for a reason. Hair everywhere helps to regulate body temperature, keeping us warm when necessary and cooler as needed. Notice that many groups from colder climates tend to be naturally hairier and those in hotter climates may have less hair, especially on the arms and legs, as the need to stay warm is not necessary. Pubic hair also helps protect the body from outside elements like dirt, aids in hydration, and may be protective against some sexually transmitted infections. Because there are nerves attached to each hair, manipulating those pubic hairs may also be pleasurable and increase sexual stimulation. Body hair is natural and helpful.

Located in the follicle are tiny sweat glands, which contribute to your signature scent. We want this hair because when your partner ventures a face (and a nose) into that area, they drink in this scent. Did you know that the organ most connected to memory formation is the nose through a part of the brain called the amygdala? There's a reason you remember the smell of your mom's cooking, which literally takes you back to those times. When a partner is exposed to your scent and the feeling is associated with pleasure, then *you* are associated with this pleasure. So why is there all this controversy regarding retaining or removing hair, especially vaginal or vulvar hair? Trends seem to come and go, and the vaginal hair pendulum swings wildly from decade to decade, and as we will discover, century to century. Along those lines, there is a rather interesting history about the removal (or non-removal) of pubic hair. It all begins as many things do, with the ancients.

In ancient Egyptian and Indian cultures, hair removal appeared to be part of daily life. Razors made of copper have been discovered and attributed to these cultures dating back to 3000 BCE. Razors have even been discovered among personal effects in the tombs of some ancient Egyptian female mummies. Ancient Egyptian and Turkish women developed something like a wax to remove hair from various parts of their bodies. Ancient Romans and Greeks were not to be left out, but their hair removal methods were somewhat more draconian. They involved tweezing out and sometimes even burning each individual hair out one by one.

Removal (or non-removal) of hair literally waxed and waned throughout the centuries. By the Elizabethan era, Queen Elizabeth I left the pubic hair but shaved the eyebrows, and that's how the high, thin brow became the fashion during that time. Fast forward to the early 20th century:

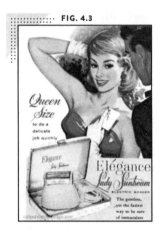

FIG. 4.3

A MCCALLS MAGAZINE AD FOR A LADIES RAZOR, CIRCA 1960.

Fashion trends changed, and by the early 1900s, smooth skin was beginning to be associated with femininity. As sleeveless dresses began to take the lead in fashion, bare armpits became the fad, and the first ads for women's razors, the Milady Décolleté, were found in *Harper's Bazaar* in 1915. Hair was characterized as "unsightly," forcing women to, of course, purchase the product. As hemlines rose and nylon shortages were instituted during World War II, hairy legs also became a no-no. All of this prepared us to go even further with shaving once the bikini was invented in 1946 and miniskirts became the rage in the 1960s.

However, in support of women's liberation, the 1970s brought freedom from shaving, and the pendulum swung back to the bush. Unfortunately, that brief respite was to be short-lived. In the late 1980s in New York City, one enterprising woman and her six sisters who immigrated from Brazil, came up with a way to remove all the hair—not just the hair on top, but the hair below. They founded a day spa where they practiced what became known as the Brazilian wax, and nothing has been the same since.

As hair removal comes and goes, so does the addition of extra hair. In some cultures, having healthy pubic hair is representative of fertility. And in the 1400s, a rather peculiar fad popped up: Since pubic lice was common (and quite itchy), many women simply shaved their hair and added a merkin, something like a vagina toupee. Sex workers of the time also found it useful to cover up any lesions or pustules that were a likely hazard of the job.[2] Even in modern times, adding hair is a trend. In modern day Korea, up to 10 percent of women suffer from a lack of pubic hair, which is called *pubic atrichosis*. Since in the Korean culture, the presence of pubic hair is seen as a sign of good health, many of those women have been known to actually get hair transplants, which can cost over two thousand dollars.[3]

As you can see, women have been experiencing controversy over whether to remove or not to remove as early as history can be told. When it comes to proper vagina care, I recommend leaving her alone and letting the bush be free. I've had a few patients ask me, "Shouldn't I shave down there because the hair will just keep growing?" No, it doesn't. Just like the hair on your head, pubic hair has a growth cycle, so it is unlikely that it will ever be long enough to braid it, unless your manual dexterity far exceeds that of the normal person. But even armed with this knowledge, I must recognize that we live in the real world, and with as much media exposure as the vagina gets on a daily basis, hair removal is here to stay. Therefore, if you choose to do so, try to avoid or at the very least minimize razor use. Why? Because razors can cause tiny nicks in the skin. Not only do those nicks increase the risk of ingrown hairs, but they can also increase the risk of sexually transmitted infections because of skin-to-skin contact. If you need to do a quick razor trim, try to wait a day or so to have sex to allow the skin to heal. And of course, you should have protected sex as an additional level of safety.

So what is the best way to remove unwanted hair?

If you must, the best way is to leave the hair at the follicle and trim the top, something like the buzz cut a new military recruit gets. An electric razor works quite nicely for this. Also, shave in the direction of the hair and try not to pull the skin taught, as that could disrupt the follicle and cause bumps. Now, you won't be bare, but there will be significantly less damage to your skin, and the glands will be left intact to support moisture and temperature. Simply put, the vagina is better when the hair is there.

WHAT ABOUT VAJACIALS OR STEAMING?

In recent years, some of my patients have asked me about the newer ways that have been invented to part you from your money, such as vajacials or steaming. They may sound reasonable, and a few patients have told me they had them with no side effects. As for benefits, I like to look for data, and there is none to prove any improvement in the state of your vagina. With a price range from $40 to $80, a vajacial is a made-up term for a vaginal facial, meaning many of the same treatments such as exfoliation, masks, and even toner are used on your vaginal skin. These treatments are supposed to somehow improve her. I say, how can one improve upon perfection? If she has soap, water, and sunshine—nothing extra is needed. Not to mention the fact that if these treatments were to cause harm, a technician would probably not be able to tell if anything is really wrong.

Another burgeoning phenomenon is vaginal steaming. Apparently, you get to sit on what looks like a medieval toilet and have a warm pot of any combination of herbs such as rosemary, mugwort, chamomile, and basil, among others, placed under your seat. This treatment is sold as a way to clean your uterus and help cure conditions such as painful menstrual cramps, fatigue, infertility, and even digestive issues. I have a very good friend who does vaginal steaming after a relationship ends as a type of ritual cleansing, fully understanding that while it may help her forget about an ex, the ritual is not a treatment for any disease other than a broken heart. Remember, your vagina (and uterus for that matter) is a self-cleaning oven, and these measures are superfluous at best. At worst, you may get burned or alter your natural pH, which could facilitate an infection. Overall, it's not worth the money or the trouble. Light some candles and have a warm bath for free.[4]

Vagina Care Do's and Don'ts

DO:

- Give her soap, water, and sunshine.
- Wear cotton underwear.
- Limit thong wear to three hours (three-hour thongs).
- Take off leggings ASAP after a workout.
- Sleep commando unless you're bleeding.
- Enjoy protected sex every time.
- Wipe from front to back.
- Clean your dildos and vaginal toys after each use.
- Recognize that your signature scent is absolutely and completely normal.
- Wear padded shorts for cycling to decrease pressure.
- Keep the hair down there.
- Use water- or silicone-based lubricant.
- Do your Kegel exercises.
- Pat her dry after a shower or bath.
- Track your vaginal bleeding patterns.
- Enjoy vaginal sex first, then anal sex second if desired (always front to back!).

DON'T:

- Sleep in underwear unless you're bleeding: see sunshine (or moonshine) above.
- Wear leggings on a long flight: warm and moist = irritative yeast.
- Urinate after sex to reduce UTI: It's never been proven to prevent one.
- Engage in anal, then vaginal sex: By bringing the e.coli from your rear to your vagina, you actually could get a UTI!
- Use oil-based lubricants like petroleum jelly or olive oil: That can put holes in condoms, and olive oil is better in pesto.

- Douche, ever, unless you're talking about the French word for a normal shower.
- Lay around in a wet bathing suit: Moisture can breed annoying yeast.
- Overuse baby wipes: They may dry your vagina and certainly won't help with pH balance.
- Steam her: That's for vegetables.
- Wear panty liners every day: No breathing, remember?
- Use feminine spray or talc-based powder: Both are irritating and possibly harmful to the skin.
- Use a loofah or shower scrunchie: It may irritate your vulva and isn't necessary to clean her any better.
- Bother with a vajacial, a "vaginal facial": If you do the aforementioned care items, you won't need it. Spend that money on a new dildo.
- Razor your vagina if you're prone to ingrown hairs: See "DO keep the hair down there."
- Put yogurt, garlic, or any other foodstuffs into your vagina: Vaginas aren't meant for salad dressing.
- Put yoni eggs or pearls in there to detoxify your vagina: She's not toxic.
- Put marijuana in there: Make brownies instead!

DID YOU KNOW?

In a 2010 study conducted among 2,000 sexually active women, 88 percent of women ages 18–24 reported removing some or all of their pubic hair.[5]

And in the 2011 movie *The Girl with the Dragon Tattoo*, actress Rooney Mara had to wear a merkin to match the hair color from the character in the book.

5

There's Something on My Vagina! (It's Probably a Mole)

I know it's been there my whole life;
I just don't like it.

—A. L., AGE 24

Removal of all the hair around the vulva and vaginal area has brought me lots of business, because women can examine the vulvar skin much more closely. But just because you now can see your vagina more clearly, it doesn't mean that bump you found is a problem. Come with me, and let us now discuss things on your vagina.

GET DOWN THERE AND LOOK

I encourage all women to take a close look at their vaginas. Each vagina is unique, and if you are familiar with the way yours looks, you can be more aware of irregularities and what you should and should *not* be concerned about, so get out a mirror. If you are examining the vulva, labia, or perineum, first look at the color of the skin. If you have darker skin, the labia minora (inner lips) themselves may be darker than the rest of your body. This is completely normal. If you are lighter skinned, the labia minora may appear pink. Little hanging flesh-colored, tag-like things are usually just that: skin tags, or the remnants of the hymen if you have engaged in penetrative sex. Also don't forget that the skin around the vagina is still skin too, and more likely than not you may have a mole or two. What you are looking for is any big change in the skin color, especially if it begins to appear much paler or much darker in one particular spot. If this is the case, bring this to a practitioner's attention.

Keep examining. Check the texture of the skin around the introitus, or vaginal opening. Often we find this skin to be somewhat less smooth, and it may have fine hair follicles but may not actually have hair growth. These are all *normal* findings. The entire female genitalia is both functional *and* beautiful—moles, tags, and all.

What else might you see? Folds! Depending on your body type, you may see a few extra folds of skin. While these are normal, if you find that you accumulate moisture in these, pay a little extra attention to your symptoms. If you are more irritated in those folds specifically, check the color of the skin. Red with small bumps and flaky skin may indicate that yeast has gotten away from the vagina and onto the skin.

WHAT DOES ABNORMAL LOOK LIKE?

What should you be concerned about? If there is one particular spot that you can always point out that is irritated, or if the color is very different from the rest, or if it's itching out of control, make sure to see your practitioner and show it to them. Just so you know, cancer of the vagina and vulva is quite rare in those under 40.

What else might be abnormal, among the things you can see? Here are a few things to take note of:

- Very pale changes in the skin
- Very dark changes in the skin

- Redness
- Flaking skin
- Swelling
- Tiny splits in the skin
- Open sores
- Growths

Very pale skin

Of course, common things happen commonly, so we are discussing the most common possible causes of a pale, itchy vagina. The first thing that springs to mind for me is atrophy. Atrophy is a result of cellular degeneration, or a gradual breakdown of healthy cells. Atrophy occurs when the estrogen levels serving the vagina drop, which can cause the skin to become pale and dry. While this may be a normal part of menopause, if it causes extreme discomfort, we would still recommend some evaluation and possible treatment, if only to make life easier. Younger women may suffer from atrophy too, in some cases. I often recommend simple emollients to start. Diaper rash cream is a good one to try, and so is nipple butter or any emollient without extra additives such as perfumes. If simple things don't help, or if the skin becomes very dark, we may want to do a biopsy to look at the cells under the microscope and make sure they aren't misbehaving (turning into cancer).

A more uncommon condition that causes pale skin and irritative itching and burning is called *lichen sclerosus*. Although we don't know exactly why or how it happens, we do know it happens in extremes of age, in both younger and older women. The medical community believes it may be autoimmune related, environmental, or even hormonal in nature. The condition looks very similar to simple atrophy but the edges can be seen more clearly. The skin may also look thicker or feel more coarse. Either of these conditions, atrophy or lichen sclerosus, will probably require some type of prescription, but sometimes topical emollients, or soaking baths of salt or colloidal oatmeal may be soothing.

Very pale vaginal skin over a large area may also be due to vitiligo. If you remember that Michael Jackson turned from Black to White, it is rumored that he had this condition that causes the melanin (which gives skin its color) to leave the skin cells due to an autoimmune disease. This condition may involve the vaginal area and labia and proceed down toward the anus, and it can be fairly itchy. In addition, there may be plaques on other places such as the elbows or face. Unfortunately, we usually treat this symptomatically as there is no cure.

Very dark skin

Darker brown skin patches may be seen in women with naturally higher melanin concentrations, which may cause the genital area to have darker skin than the rest of the body. If it is not itchy, we call this normal. The color may also intensify with pregnancy and can be responsive to hormones, both of which are completely normal changes. However, if you do start to get an itchy vagina and your thighs rub together when you walk, check the skin. Does it feel different in that area? Does the skin feel thick or look like cowhide? Depending on our weight and what we wear, these changes often occur from friction. If you're a leggings girl, scale back on tight-fitting clothing. If you're a heavy girl, pay attention to how the legs rub together and consider a mild cream (over the counter hydrocortisone is probably OK) to help decrease friction. Of course, if you're still itching, it's always best to be checked out by a pro.

Redness

Redness, or erythema, when seen with an itchy vagina, is most commonly a sign of inflammation. Inflammation can come from multiple places: infection, environment, shaving and waxing, rubbing or trauma, and so on. If it's short-lived and goes away on its own, then you're probably fine. Eczema is a common cause of this minor annoyance and can be seriously, raging-yeast-infection itchy. If you already have asthma or skin conditions like eczema, it's actually more common and should be one of the first things you think about. However, if it stays red and becomes warm, then it's time to be seen.

Flaking skin

Most of the time, it's just a sign that she's dry! We spend a lot of time removing things from her but forget that she may need a bit of primping herself to keep the vaginal skin healthy and moisturized. Again, a fragrance-free moisturizer will be your friend here.

Psoriasis is another bothersome but not necessarily dangerous condition that can occur on the vulva and in other places, resulting in an itchy vagina. Watch out for red and flaky skin and a shiny, scaly appearance. Psoriasis is autoimmune-related and will generally require a doctor's care. Another possible condition that causes red, flaky skin is *tinea cruris*, also known as jock itch. Men aren't the only ones who can get a yeast infection of the skin. Look for tiny itchy bumps immediately outside the area of flaky skin.

Swelling

There could be a lot of things going on here. Some of the more common conditions are again just infection, trauma, and so on. I once had a patient who experienced severe vaginal swelling from her new career as a spin instructor. However, there are a few pesky sexually transmitted infections that one may also consider such as chlamydia or gonorrhea. If you get the triple-threat of swelling, redness, AND pain, then skip the ice packs and get thee to the doctor.

Tiny splits

Sometimes itching and scratching of the vagina can become the condition itself. When we tell you not to scratch, we mean it! You could develop a condition called *lichen simplex chronicus*, which results from too much itching, scratching, and rubbing. You get yourself into what we call an "itch-scratch cycle." Your skin can become thick and rough, and it can sometimes lose some sensation, and who likes that? If you find that these splits come and go, it may be something entirely different, like a herpes infection. Monitor this closely, and get tested if this symptom seems to repeat.

Sores

Unfortunately, sores are almost never normal. The most common sore-causing condition is herpes. There are a couple of types, but suffice it to say that either type can cause very painful sores that come and go over a lifetime. It's most contagious just before an outbreak or just at the outset of one, so you may not notice anything on a lover. In addition, there is NO cure, only treatment that may reduce the frequency of episodes or treat the symptoms of an active flare-up.

Another sore-causing condition that is a bit rarer but also sexually transmitted is called *lymphogranuloma venereum*. Sounds terrible, I know, and it is! It's caused by chlamydia. If you don't live in a tropical region, however, this is lower on your list of worries.

Growths

Growths are certainly a thing to get examined. If you feel something raised on your vaginal area, have a look. This is simply the best way to start. We clinicians organize these by color, then shape, then texture. Read on for information about various colors. Keep in mind, some conditions may fit into several categories; color will vary with skin tone, so it's best to let a doctor determine what's going on.

Little red spots

We often think, especially if accompanied by severe itching and red, flaky skin, these may be indicative of a yeast infection of the skin itself as we discussed before. Now, if you just see scattered red spots, which may be a little raised or even flat, these are usually benign growths called *cherry hemangiomas*. These are simply a collection of capillaries and blood vessels. They may not be confined to the vagina and can occur anywhere else on the body, usually the trunk. Although they may increase during pregnancy, these little guys are usually not of concern.

Flesh-colored

The most common type of flesh-colored growth I see in my office is the simple ingrown hair bump. The technical term is *pseudofolliculitis*, and it occurs most often after shaving. The cure? Don't shave, or have the hair lasered off, so no hair at all grows to cause the bump. The treatment? I usually recommend warm compresses, sitz baths (lukewarm baths with baking soda), and loose-fitting clothing. It will usually resolve on its own. If it persists longer than a few weeks, have your gyno take a look.

If your growth looks as if someone "stuck" it there and has the appearance of a tiny cauliflower, one of the first things on the list of what it could be is genital warts. Caused by HPV, the human papilloma virus, warts come from skin-to-skin contact and are quite contagious, especially if the contact is with an active wart. These firm, irregularly rough growths are usually skin-colored, but they can also be red, brown, pink, white, or tan. The change in color is due to overgrowth and thickening of the affected cells from being in a moist location such as the vaginal area.

Growths that are a little more hang-y could simply be skin tags. They are essentially flesh-colored moles, and while they may cause discomfort, they are not dangerous.

If you see small, round, shiny dome-shaped growths that have a tiny indentation in the middle like a belly button with your itch, it could be a condition called *molluscum contagiosum*. While it is NOT a sexually transmitted infection, it comes from a virus that comes from, as we say, "close personal contact." Because this virus is in the same family as chicken pox, it can also proliferate in places like schools where there are many small children (not in the genital area, though). In adults, however, it tends to occur around the vagina or genital area and cause itching.

After having a baby, the place where the vagina tore (or was cut) and was repaired and healed can form a scar, which can be raised, itchy, irregular, and overall uncomfortable. I've seen many patients who suffer with chronic itching and scarring after having a baby, and it can be a frustrating and difficult thing to contend with. Some treatments can include massaging the area (really), injections, or topical steroid creams like hydrocortisone. Depending on how bad the scar is, it may also need to be revised with surgery.

Blue/black

If you see anything on the vagina that is blue or black and itchy, look closely. Examine the borders. Does it look smooth or irregular? Is it branching out or spreading? If it looks strange, then see your doctor. When you're looking at a spot with regular borders and uniform color, 90 percent of the time it's just a mole and you can leave it alone. It could also be varicose veins or little breaks in the blood vessels that simply occur with being alive and putting weight on the vagina or with pregnancy (you're seeing a trend here, yes?).

Yellow

Depending on the amount of melanin in your skin, any of the things described above may appear yellow or paler, almost white. Does it feel smooth or rough? A note to remember: If it's rough, it probably came from an outside source. Smooth things tend to come from within ourselves, growing from under the skin. Various cysts spring to my mind, the most common of which is a smooth cyst called an *epidermal inclusion cyst*. These are a collection of keratin (protein found in hair and nails) deposits and can range from the size of the head of a pin, called milia, to much larger, hard inclusions sometimes the size of a walnut or bigger. The presence of keratin is why they may feel hard to the touch. I usually leave these things alone unless they start to cause itching or discomfort.

Now that you've looked closely at your vagina, how can you really tell the difference between all these things? I'm just giving guidelines here. Occasionally, looking alone may not give us the diagnosis or even a hint at one. If this is the case, your doctor/practitioner may actually have to take a tiny piece of your skin to be examined under the microscope. The cells will usually give us the answer, and we can take it from there.

DID YOU KNOW?

Of the more than 150 types of HPV we can be exposed to, only two of these, types 6 and 11, cause nearly all genital warts.[1]

6

My Vagina Is Itchy and It Burns!

What do you mean it's the thong?
—C. S., AGE 29

The most common reason for a woman to visit the gynecologist is vaginitis. The term *vaginitis* is a bit of a catch-all phrase that can include a multitude of conditions. The annoying itchiness, burning, redness, and pain that brings you to my door is most often from a simple yeast infection. Of course, there are other, much more serious conditions that we will touch upon, but first let's focus our attention on this common condition and what we can do to alleviate and even prevent it.

THE DREADED YEAST INFECTION

Yeast is a common type of fungus that lives everywhere in and on our bodies. There are many types of yeast, but the one that affects us most frequently is called *Candida albicans* (*C. albicans*). *C. albicans* is not the only species from the *Candida* family that lives in the body. Other common species include *C. glabrata*, *C. parapsilosis*, *C. tropicalis*, and *C. krusei*. These five species of yeast cause over 90 percent of all vaginal yeast infections.

Under normal circumstances, yeast does no harm. However, for some women, yeast can morph into invasive forms and penetrate into the vaginal and vulvar tissue; this results in a painful condition known as *yeast vaginitis* or *vulvovaginal candidiasis* (VVC).

VVC is the second most common form of vaginitis. The symptoms of VVC are itching, burning, generalized vulvar pain, painful sex, pain with urination, discharge, redness, and swelling. Persistent itching of the vulva/labia that does not respond to normal hygienic measures (like changing damp underwear or showering more frequently) could be the result of VVC. VVC is similar to jock itch in males and is very painful. The VVC discharge (if present) is thick and white, yellow, or occasionally green in color, sometimes described as cottage-cheese-like, and may smell like rising dough (which, of course, is full of yeast). VVC is NOT the result of sexually transmitted diseases or poor hygiene. However, intercourse is a source of moisture and heat, both of which contribute to the risk of developing this particularly itchy type of vagina, especially if the vagina is not aired out accordingly. Remember, she loves to breathe.

Recipe for a Yeast Infection

- 1 thong
- 1 panty liner (thong-sized, of course)
- 1 pair of tights
- 1 skinny jean or legging
- Take any combination of these and mix together for 2 days.

The risk factors for developing yeast are excessive warmth, moisture, antibiotic exposure, receptive oral sex, hot tubs, frequent sexual intercourse, spermicides, pregnancy, hormonal contraception, diabetes, immunosuppression, estrogen deficiency or excess, chemical douches, exercise (heat and moisture), tight-fitting clothes, warmer climates, and other vaginal conditions like bacterial vaginosis that can alter the pH of the vagina. The picture below is of yeast "buds" on the left and "hyphae" on the right. The hyphae shapes cause the infection whereas the buds are dormant. Interestingly, 70 percent of women carry yeast buds in their vaginas but not all of those women get a yeast infection.[1]

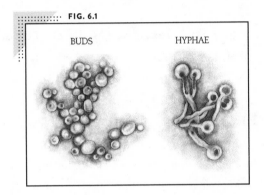

FIG. 6.1

BUDS   HYPHAE

YEAST BUDS (LEFT) AND HYPHAE (RIGHT).

How do I prevent a yeast infection? (Hint: Don't wear thongs.)

A question I often get in my office is how do you reduce your chances of getting a yeast infection? As we said, most women are carriers of the buds, and the balance that exists among the healthy bacteria (*Lactobacilli*), bad bacteria (often *Gardnerella*), and yeast is very delicate. At least twice a day, I diagnose someone complaining of an itchy vagina with VVC, and they often have something in common: They wear leggings or a thong daily. The fatal flaw is leggings after the gym or leggings *and* a thong (the absolute kiss of yeast for sure). Imagine the warmth and moisture that comes from either of those, and you have an automatic recipe for those yeast cells to go from dormant to active. I understand that thongs are popular, but as I tell my patients, they are three-hour underwear. Wear them out on a date or any other necessarily underwear-minimizing event, then remove immediately thereafter to minimize the possibility of yeast conversion and that itchy vagina.

Interestingly enough, thong underwear was never meant to be worn all day. As legend goes, it was invented during the 1939 World's Fair when New York's Mayor LaGuardia decreed that all-nude dancers had to cover up certain areas. Instead of completely covering up, the dancers donned thongs, which covered just enough to pass muster by the apparently prudish mayor.[2]

How do I treat a yeast infection? (Hint: Don't douche.)

Currently, the treatment of VVC consists of over-the-counter (OTC) creams such as miconazole (otherwise known as Monistat™) or an oral antifungal prescribed by a healthcare practitioner, such as fluconazole. Miconazole is effective in about 50–70 percent of VVC cases. In some cases, vulvar burning and pain increase after miconazole application and continues for the next several days because miconazole breaks open the yeast cell wall, which releases toxic contents that inflame the already very sensitive vaginal skin before it eventually heals. This is why sometimes your vagina gets itchier before it feels better.

If using miconazole is your only option, the best time to use the cream or suppository is at night. The medication sticks better if you're lying down for that extended period of time. If you use it in the morning, consider inserting a tampon to keep the ingredients inside so that the chemicals do not spill out of your vagina and sting the external genitalia. It can also take a few days to feel relief. In the meantime, to stop the symptoms of pain, itching, or swelling, try putting frozen peas or frozen corn (or your chosen vegetable-du-jour, but probably not broccoli or a veggie with sharper edges) in a plastic bag, cover it with a damp washcloth, and apply the cold pack to the vulva for about fifteen minutes. This can act as a temporary soothing measure if things get really annoying.

Some over-the-counter medications can contain chemicals that numb the area temporarily and can help your itchy vagina symptoms but do nothing to cure the infectious forms of yeast found in VVC. These tempering measures are ultimately unhelpful as the true underlying problem is not addressed, and you just spent money on something that doesn't work. When the symptoms return, repeat applications, delays in proper treatment, and confusion occur.

Douching is absolutely ineffective against any form of vaginitis and is considered an utterly useless, unsafe practice by the American College of Obstetricians and Gynecologists. Why unsafe? Because what if it's something more serious like a sexually transmitted infection and it goes untreated? Just stop by and get checked.

In addition, douching can often result in an increase in unhealthy bacteria because fluid and chemicals flush and disrupt the vagina's delicate ecosystem or microbiome and throw off the pH balance, killing the wonderful happy (*Lactobacillus*) bacteria. Once harmful bacteria gain control, they can be very difficult to eradicate, even with medication, because the healthy bacteria need to again gain a foothold in the eternal battle for the vaginal milieu. And with douching, there is the risk of pushing harmful bacteria such as gonorrhea and chlamydia into the uterus and fallopian tubes, which increases the risk of pelvic inflammatory disease (PID). One episode of PID is enough to cause fallopian tubes to be blocked or scarred in up to 15 percent of women, leading to *tubal factor* infertility. Once blocked, the sperm and egg cannot meet, or if a sperm does get through, a fertilized egg gets stuck in the tube causing an ectopic or tubal pregnancy, which can be life-threatening. There is no point in douching *ever*, with these risks.

If you find yourself at your gynecologist for treatment of itching and burning, you will likely be prescribed fluconazole (brand name Diflucan), the most popular yeast infection medication. It is an oral medication that must be prescribed by a physician, nurse practitioner, or PA. Fluconazole is about 70 percent effective and takes about 36–48 hours to take full effect.

The problem with oral medications is that the drugs go into the bloodstream and may affect all organs. They have risks and side effects that could be harmful, such as making the yeast resistant to current antifungal drugs. Avoiding this resistance is critical in the immunocompromised population, such as those with HIV, because a blood infection from *Candida albicans* can be fatal up to 40 percent of the time. So I actually try a vaginal antifungal before jumping to any pills taken by mouth.

Over-the-counter intravaginal agents

- Clotrimazole 1% cream 5 g intravaginally daily for 7–14 days
- Clotrimazole 2% cream 5 g intravaginally daily for 3 days
- Miconazole 2% cream 5 g intravaginally daily for 7 days
- Miconazole 4% cream 5 g intravaginally daily for 3 days
- Miconazole 100 mg vaginal suppository, one suppository daily for 7 days
- Miconazole 200 mg vaginal suppository, one suppository daily for 3 days
- Miconazole 1,200 mg vaginal suppository, one suppository for 1 day
- Tioconazole 6.5% ointment 5 g intravaginally in a single application

Prescription intravaginal agents

- Butoconazole 2% cream (single-dose bio-adhesive product), 5 g intravaginally in a single application
- Terconazole 0.4% cream 5 g intravaginally daily for 7 days
- Terconazole 0.8% cream 5 g intravaginally daily for 3 days
- Terconazole 80 mg vaginal suppository, one suppository daily for 3 days[3]

Topical "azoles" are very effective against *C. albicans*, but not as effective against other *Candida* species. These beast yeasts are often treated with other antifungal medications such as amphotericin B (Abelcet, AmBisome, Amphocin, Amphotec, or Fungizone), flucytosine, or nystatin (Mycostatin). My patients with itchy vaginas will often show up after multiple courses of over-the-counter "azole" medications, but when we test, they show up with *C. glabrata*, *C. krusei*, or some other type of yeast that needs a different antifungal. If your vagina is unhappy with itching and burning and over-the-counters don't help, it is imperative to go see a practitioner, as you may be treating yourself wrong. It could be something different altogether too, so don't wait.[4]

Do natural remedies work?

There are many alternative options for treating yeast vaginitis. Some of these natural therapies may help and others are likely not worth your money. Many of these have roots in science and history, but some do not. I understand it may be tempting to try these, but before you put anything in there, I encourage you to do the research and get the real data.

From *The Trotula* (12th-century gynecologic text):

If there is itching in the vagina,
take camphor, litharge, laurel berry,
and egg white and let a pessary be made.
Galen says a powder of fenugreek
or goose tallow is good . . .[5]

Alternative treatments for yeast have literally been around since antiquity as we can see from our medieval text, but although camphor may be an effective treatment, I'm sure that it cannot have been comfortable. Fenugreek powder or goose tallow may be a little soothing, but they most likely will not cure yeast. In addition, many costly treatments you can find may not be as effective as they tout themselves to be, and their promises for a healthy, happy vagina may not ever be kept. Here's a short list of things that my patients have used for their itchy vaginas; let's address them one by one and see what works, what doesn't, and which ones cause the biggest mess!

Greek yogurt: probably useful

Aside from the obvious mess and the fact that you could simply be eating it, putting yogurt in the vagina is probably not going to cause any long-term damage. However, if you don't want Yoplait in your panties, check out this interesting study from Egypt in 2017.[6] They studied two hundred women with a confirmed diagnosis of vaginal yeast infection and had them eat one cup of plain unsweetened yogurt every day for two weeks while treating their infections with a routine antifungal. What they found was that eating the yogurt resulted in an increase in *Lactobacillus acidophilus* as well as a real decrease in symptoms. Just to compare, those who did not eat the dose of yogurt every day had more complaints of yeast than those who ate the yogurt. So, don't insert, just indulge.

Boric acid: useful, but dangerous

Yes, it does sound scary, and it actually is. For routine yeast infections, boric acid should not be used. It can actually cause some serious damage (or even kill you) if you accidentally ingest it. Now, if you have one of the other species of yeast that we previously discussed, meaning one that's NOT *Candida albicans*, and it is resistant to virtually everything else, this is the only case that this potentially dangerous formula should be used under the direction of a clinician. Oh, and the dose is 600mg vaginally for two weeks. No thank you, if there are other options.

Hydrogen peroxide: probably not useful

We know that in a healthy vagina, the good bacteria, our friend *Lactobacillus*, makes lactic acid and hydrogen peroxide, which helps maintain a good pH balance in the bacteria, so it sounds like a great idea to douche with peroxide, doesn't it? Don't do it. If we want our vaginas to remain in balance, adding a whopping dose (yes, even the 3 percent from drugstore peroxide is whopping) to your vagina could easily throw off your balance and result in little else other than irritation. While it may be soothing to add some to a bath, it is certainly not helpful to douche. Ever.

Oil of oregano: maybe useful

In this instance, wild oregano specifically was studied, and the studies I've found tend to be lab studies. This means we don't have enough information to say that this will really cure a yeast infection in an actual person. A few other cooking ingredients have been studied as well: thyme, marjoram, mint, cinnamon, salvia, and clove. So if delicious is what you're looking for, then use them for cooking, but for itchy vagina yeast, these are probably a no. Oil of oregano is also a natural blood thinner, so if you're anemic or have a bleeding or clotting disorder, just avoid it. It may also reduce blood sugar, so diabetics should also be careful if you're dealing with the concentrated oil. Also, keep in mind that all oil-based formulas weaken condoms, making safer sex a real problem.[7]

Garlic: maybe useful

Eat, don't insert! Garlic contains a compound called allicin that contains antifungal properties. Allicin is only found when garlic is chewed or crushed. And again, we only have lab studies thus far, nothing in humans. Therefore, sticking a clove in there will only ward off vampires.[8]

Coconut oil: probably not useful

Again, yummy, but so-so on vagina yeast. What science has found out so far is that it can be useful in oral *Candida* infections in small children and in the lab. There has not been a single study anywhere about using coconut oil for vaginal yeast. So it's probably OK to try if you want to explore, but be aware that oils reduce condom effectiveness, and if you're using it for weeks on end and don't feel any better, have someone (not just your partner) check it out.[9]

Apple cider vinegar: probably not useful

Apple cider vinegar is good for salads, not for douching. It has antibacterial and antifungal properties that have been proven (again, just in the lab, not in humans). If you feel like you want to try it, think about adding a bit to a bath (no douching ever, remember?), because the concentrated product could burn and basically kill all your vaginal bacteria—good, bad, and ugly—not to mention increase your risk for other vaginal infections. The study I found also discovered that apple cider vinegar didn't even work that well for *Candida*, the most common form of itchy vagina yeast.[10]

Gentian violet: useful

The original synthesis of this 19th-century remedy has been attributed to French chemist Charles Lauth in 1861, who gave it the name "Violet de Paris." Historically, it was marketed as a cure-all, from bacterial infections to ulcers to cancer. Gentian violet was first found to be useful against *Candida* in 1912, and it has enjoyed a resurgence in the 21st century because bacteria and fungal organisms have developed resistance against modern treatments. The biggest drawback is the violet. It is incredibly staining. So if you're interested in channeling Prince, and it's permanently stained purple underwear you want, go for it. Use for 10–14 days as a treatment for itching and yeast.[11]

Tea tree oil: maybe useful

Tea tree oil is an extract from a plant found in Australia. Again, the only studies that seem to support its use come from the lab, which suggest that it may be an effective antifungal. However, putting this very strong oil into your vagina could actually damage the delicate tissue (and it really burns). And, it really has a rather interesting, medicinal smell that may put off even the most eager of lovers, not to mention that thing about oil and condoms. If you must, think about adding a few drops to a bath.[12]

Probiotics: maybe useful

Probiotics have been touted as a way to keep your intestinal tract healthy. Because research has shown that there are healthy bacteria in our guts that impact our overall health, a probiotic may not be a bad idea.[13] Unfortunately, there are so many products out there, and since they are marketed as dietary supplements and aren't regulated, it's tough to figure out which one will help you the most. A probiotic containing at least *Lactobacillus* must be taken daily and on a long-term basis to get the best effect. What I've discovered is that many of my patients will take any given regimen for about a week, and if it doesn't work immediately, they give up. Give any new probiotic at least a month. Keep in mind that probiotics aren't antibiotics. The "pro" part of the biotic means you're building something up, and if you've ever watched a building being demolished you know it takes longer to build than to destroy. Additionally, many over-the-counters contain the wrong species of *Lactobacillus*, and most strains are deactivated when passing through the stomach and natural acids of the gut. Take-home message: Take any supplement to your doc and let them have a look.

Do antibiotics cause yeast infections?

In order to address the myth that taking almost any antibiotic causes a woman to get an itchy vagina due to a yeast infection, we must look at the data. According to the *British Medical Journal*, only 18–24 percent of women who take antibiotics will get a yeast infection. Also, keep in mind that the antibiotics that resulted in the most yeast infections were the heavy-duty ones, the "broad spectrum" antibiotics that kill most anything. So if you got a little amoxicillin for an ear infection or were treated for a simple urinary tract infection at the urgent care center, the likelihood that you'll need to call us for a resultant yeast infection is only 24 percent. So before you reach for that Monistat, give it a day, stop wearing leggings and/or thong underwear, and let your itchy vagina simply rest and breathe. She'll thank you for it.[14]

VULVODYNIA

In some cases, itching and burning may not have anything to do with an infection. Many patients I have seen have been treated by multiple doctors with multiple courses of antifungals, tried all sorts of yogurt and tea tree oil, and have not gotten better at all. In this case, other culprits besides your run-of-the-mill itchy vagina yeast infection must be considered, even some of the more serious ones.

I had a patient, not too long ago, who came to me with persistent itching and burning. We checked for routine conditions such as sexually transmitted infections and (of course) examined for yeast. She had nothing of the sort. I was also the third physician she had seen about this, and she was beginning to become desperate. Her relationship with her boyfriend was strained because she was reticent to have sex due to the burning, and she was at her wit's end. She had tried both over-the-counter and prescription medications with only short-term improvement. She noticed burning when merely sitting down. Her work was even beginning to be affected. When the itching and burning become so severe that it affects your life and nothing seems to help, there are other conditions that we have to think about. We worked together and found her diagnosis: vulvodynia.

By definition, vulvodynia is defined as a chronically irritated vagina and vulvar pain and burning of unknown cause after having investigated and ruled out all other conditions including cancer. We find it across the age spectrum. Vulvodynia affects approximately 3–15 percent of women and has no known cause. The burning and itching can be debilitating, worse when sitting, and may have come from a previous trauma, infection, inflammation, or autoimmune cause. Note: It's probably *not* your hormones. Women on hormonal birth control seem to be no more or less affected than others. Unfortunately, women's health is not well researched and the information we have is limited. Therefore, I will present what science knows and what seems to help from our experience, and what we ultimately did to help this patient.

I was able to diagnose her after she came back for the third time complaining of yeast infection symptoms. Previously, she really did have yeast, albeit a small amount. We treated her symptoms as if she had a yeast infection, and she improved. However, I started to become suspicious. I took a little cotton swab and brushed the vulvar area. She didn't like that. This is called the cotton swab test. Unaffected vaginas will only feel a cotton swab, but those vaginas suffering from vulvodynia will feel pinprick-like burning pain. Now, this test is not 100 percent reliable, but it certainly helps to point us in the right direction.

Treating vulvodynia

When tackling such a persistent itchy vagina and burning like that of vulvodynia, we run through a long list of treatments for this chronic issue. In addition to topical treatments like numbing cream or lidocaine for occasional flares, we encourage all of our patients with this annoying condition to see a pelvic floor therapist. What we have learned about pelvic floor therapy and about vulvodynia in general is that it appears the nerves become overactive and need to be downregulated or calmed down. In this way, the pain and burning can be diminished.

A few other treatments have proven successful. Some of them are quite simple, and others, well—they involve a bit more:

- Take a lukewarm bath with baking soda. It's called a sitz bath, taken from the German *sitzen*, literally "to sit." It can soothe those overactive nerves.

- Change your detergent fragrance-free or even use a detergent made for babies.

- Try topical creams, including anti-inflammatories like cortisone, numbing creams such as lidocaine (careful if using before sex; you could make your partner's genitals numb too!), or estrogen cream in perimenopausal and menopausal vaginas.

- Avoid binding clothing. When your vagina can't breathe, the nerves get angry and retaliate against you, causing burning and pain.

- Try acupuncture. There is a growing body of evidence that is supportive of trying acupuncture as an adjunct to Western methods.

A 2019 review from the Society of Korean Medicine Obstetrics and Gynecology stated that acupuncture was effective at treating vulvar pain and associated sexual pain and improving quality of life. Hey, two thousand-plus years of knowledge and experience can't be that wrong, no? Remember, we respect alternative treatments with evidence, so it may be worth a go.[15]

- Make dietary changes. A quick Google search on relieving vulvar pain with diet will give you something called a "low-oxalate" diet. This came from a single study in 1991 that showed that a single patient had high oxalates in her urine. Although we have since proven that not all patients with vulvodynia or any other pain syndrome have high oxalates, this diet seems to be popular. Food high in oxalates include spinach, rhubarb, bran flakes, and nut butters.[16]

- Medications might work. There are several on the market, all of which have some level of scientific support, such as amitriptyline, pregabalin, gabapentin, or duloxetine.

- Biofeedback is a mind-body technique used to allow you to control your perception of certain sensations and involuntary bodily functions. Sensors are placed at various points on your body and connected to an EEG device that measures brain waves. Working with a therapist for thirty- to sixty-minute sessions, you progressively learn to downregulate your pain sensors.

- Nerve blocks are sometimes an option. Usually performed by an anesthesiologist or a trained gynecologist, this technique literally blocks the conduction of nerve fibers with the injection of a local anesthetic. Of course, this is temporary and used in some of the most extreme cases.

- Surgery is our last-ditch effort. Usually used for pinpoint or provoked vulvodynia, we actually remove the vestibular glands. Success can be as high as 90 percent, but this is, of course, reserved for those who do not respond to any of our other efforts.

You may be wondering how I ended up helping my patient. Well, we did a combination of topical lidocaine and gabapentin, which after lots of trial and error seems to help her best. We also armed her with the knowledge that the condition is likely chronic, that it's NOT her fault, and that we may need to adjust our approach over time.

If this sounds like you, and your vagina is still itchy and burning after using over-the-counter meds over and over, as a savvy vagina owner, don't self-diagnose—have a pro take a look.[17]

Itchy Vagina FAQs

- **Why does my vagina itch/burn?** Aside from the conditions discussed in detail here, some of the main culprits are the things we do to her ourselves! If you use any of the following (this list is not exhaustive but will give you the gist), itching can result:

  - Scented soaps
  - Bubble baths
  - Feminine sprays
  - Douches
  - Spermicides
  - Detergents
  - Fabric softeners
  - Scented toilet paper/scented wipes

  Avoid these things if you can, especially douching, smelly soaps, and using perfume in that area. This is paramount. She will usually clean up after herself, and adding extra stuff just gums up the works and makes for a more confused (and still itchy) vagina. Adding extra chemicals could throw off any possibility of achieving a natural balance, making her retaliate against you with an even more miserable itch.

- **What should I do if she starts to itch and I can't get to the doctor?**
First of all, fight the urge to scratch! Remember that scratching can
beget itching and itching begets scratching, and then you're sitting
around all weekend hot and bothered, and not in a good way. Temporary fixes include cold packs, baking soda, or oatmeal baths. If you're
not better in a few days, then make time to see the doc.

- **Is it just me or do other women have this problem?** It's certainly
not just you! Vaginal itching is more common than the common cold,
and it usually means nothing. If you've ever lived with a man, look
how often he scratches or adjusts his balls and doesn't give it a second
thought. Since we as women have been programmed to believe any
tiny itch or discomfort is bad and requires attention, we unfortunately over-diagnose ourselves, seeking remedies when there may
not be a real problem.

- **How can I tell if there's a real problem?** Occasional itching that
goes away is nothing to worry about. Itching that lasts more than a
few days or that wakes you from sleep could be a problem. If your
itch doesn't improve with the simple home remedies we talked about,
or if you see color changes, swelling, or have pain and severe burning,
see a practitioner for further investigation and more answers.

- **How can I prevent itching in the first place?** There are a few things
within your power that can keep her itch-free. Start with three easy
steps: soap, water, and sunshine.

  - Soap. Use a plain, unscented soap, hypoallergenic if you can.
  There's no need to spend extra money on special vagina soaps.
  It's really just soap.

  - Water. No need to douche. Water from the bath or shower is all
  she actually needs. Pat dry. Avoid rubbing too. That can annoy
  her skin.

  - Sunshine. Avoid all the leggings and thongs that you can. If you
  must wear them, peel them off the moment you get a chance.

DID YOU KNOW?

In 17th-century England, women were known to knead dough between their legs before baking bread to gain the love of the man who would eat it. Probably gave them a heck of a yeast infection, too.[18]

7

My Vagina Smells and There's Something Coming Out!

My vagina smells like sweat.

—THEM

Yes, that happens when you suffocate her with leggings and thong underwear. Vaginas sweat too!

—ME

The most common reason to come to the gynecologist, even more than yeast infections, is a smelly vagina with something coming out of it, and although the vast majority of discharge is normal, the most common cause for pathologic vaginal discharge is bacterial vaginosis (BV).

BV is *not* a sexually transmitted disease but tends to occur after becoming sexually active. Some risk factors include multiple sexual partners, douching, and using oil-based lubricants. Remember, oil and vinegar are for salads. The exact cause is unknown, but it appears that it's a smelly-vagina self-fulfilling prophecy. Sexual intercourse can alter the vaginal pH by increasing it slightly from basic (higher pH) sperm. Bacteria such as *Gardnerella* proliferate in an environment low in oxygen with an elevated pH. The normal, physiologic pH of the vagina is low or acidic due to the production of tiny amounts of hydrogen peroxide by the *Lactobacillus* bacteria. Therefore, the abnormal bacteria that enjoy a high pH environment, which can be facilitated by the presence of sperm, may proliferate. But why does this not happen every time you have sex? Science doesn't yet know, and because it's a woman problem, we may never find out.

Biofilms are common in both BV and yeast. These are slimy films or membranes similar to tooth scum that form in the vagina (I know, disgusting). Biofilms trap the bacteria and their waste products to produce a foul, fishy odor and discharge, that something coming out. Sometimes women will not notice anything or maybe just a smelly vagina that can become particularly pungent after sex when the semen reacts with the by-products of the bacteria. Irritation from the discharge is a common complaint, but true pain or itching is uncommon unless a yeast infection is also present. BV can make one more prone to a yeast infection because of the pH changes that yeast like to live in.

How is BV diagnosed? Your doctor or practitioner can use a few different modalities to diagnose this incredibly annoying smelly vagina condition. Most practitioners will use certain criteria, called Amsel's criteria, right in the office to diagnose it. Three of the following are usually present for diagnosis of BV:

- Homogeneous, thin, grayish-white discharge that smoothly coats the vaginal walls. Sometimes it even "pools" in the back of the vagina.
- Vaginal pH > 4.5.
- Positive "whiff test," defined as the presence of a fishy odor when a drop of 10 percent potassium hydroxide (KOH) is added to a sample of vaginal discharge. Yes, that fishy odor you may detect can actually be a thing!
- Clue cells on a saline wet mount. Clue cells are vaginal epithelial cells (skin cells) studded with adherent *coccobacilli* (bacteria) that are best visualized under a microscope at the edge of the cell. For a positive

result, at least 20 percent of the epithelial cells on the wet mount should be clue cells. The presence of clue cells diagnosed by an experienced microscopist is the single most reliable predictor of BV.[1]

Clue cells (epithelial cells coated with thousands of bacteria) are present with BV, as seen in the following image. Epithelial cells are the normal cells of the vagina's surface, seen on the left.

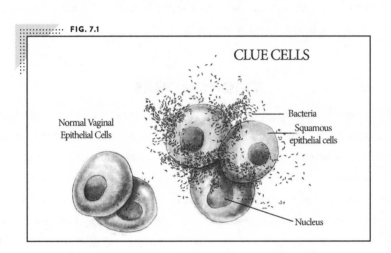

FIG. 7.1

CLUE CELLS

Normal Vaginal
Epithelial Cells

Bacteria

Squamous
epithelial cells

Nucleus

ILLUSTRATION OF A NORMAL VAGINAL CELL COMPARED WITH
ONE AFFLICTED WITH BACTERIAL VAGINOSIS.

There is also an in-office test that offers nearly instant results without using Amsel's criteria. It capitalizes on the presence of the biofilms we previously discussed made by the bad bacteria, monitors the pH, and produces a color change when BV is present.

There are some over-the-counter color change agents that are available to purchase that can easily run over 20 bucks each. But here's a hint: Save money and buy some litmus paper. Litmus paper is the basis for measuring pH and is an inexpensive way to check your own vaginal fluid if you think your vagina is getting a bit smelly. If the litmus paper turns blue, an indication of an elevated pH, it supports a diagnosis of BV.

Drugs such as metronidazole and clindamycin, both oral and topical, are the mainstay of treatment for BV. Retreatment is often necessary, so don't think there's something wrong if you need more than one course. Recent studies show that lesbian partners of women with BV usually develop an identical type of vaginal microflora. In heterosexual couples, the man often has the identical bacteria on their penis and scrotum as the woman with BV. This does not mean it is sexually transmitted. It just means that people tend to develop similar bacterial flora to those with whom they are in close bodily contact.

TRICHOMONAS

Of course, bacterial vaginosis isn't the only cause of a smelly vagina with abnormal stuff coming out of it. Another cause is trichomonas, which actually *is* a sexually transmitted infection. Trichomonas can be asymptomatic but can cause a majorly smelly vagina, which may also be paired with burning, itching, frequent urination, or painful urination. Trichomonas is not a bacterium; it's a parasite. Yes, a parasite; it is a tiny living organism that only humans host. It is pear-shaped and has four little tails, or flagella, that allow it to move. In addition to clue cells, this is another thing that doctors look for on a wet mount, an exam we can perform with a microscope to look for those pesky critters:

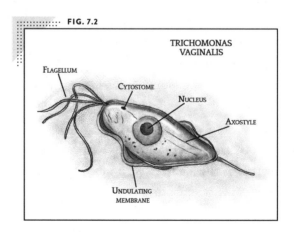

FIG. 7.2

TRICHOMONAS VAGINALIS

FLAGELLUM

CYTOSTOME

NUCLEUS

AXOSTYLE

UNDULATING MEMBRANE

Traditional medical treatment is exactly the same as for BV, which is a good thing in case trichomonas was missed in the testing but you got treated for bacterial vaginosis. You will want to tell your partners and get tested to make sure that little bugger is gone so you don't get infected again.

WHAT ELSE COULD IT BE?

I often have patients who visit me complaining of multiple episodes of odor and discharge. They're at their wit's end, and of course have tried everything you can find on the internet, both on and inside their vaginas. Some good news: For the most part, occasional odor is actually OK. Remember, as you are a dynamic organism with shifting bacteria, changing hormones, and varied diet, it's no wonder your personal vaginal smell will change. Try this: If you think your vagina is too smelly, drink a good two liters of water. If that doesn't flush the smell in a day or so, then schedule an appointment with your gynecologist and get checked. Also, keep in mind it is completely normal for the vagina to have a mild, musky smell. This odor can change with hormonal shifts during menstruation, pregnancy, and menopause. A subtle smell is not a cause for concern. Consider it your "signature scent."

It's smelly

Wearing leggings and thongs can cause a little odor, but a little odor may actually be normal. Certain bacteria on the skin may have a little smell if you get sweaty or warm. Also, certain foods when consumed in a large enough quantity can affect the odor of your vagina. Think beer and a yeasty smell without an actual yeast infection.

Here we have broken down some of the most common vagina smells, including their how's and why's:

Fish fillet

You've probably heard an abnormal vaginal odor described as fishy. This misnomer has been used to describe vaginas in a derogatory way for decades. In fact, actual fresh fish doesn't smell like too much of anything. Truth be told, decomposing fish is the more reasonable comparison. I know that doesn't sound much better. But why is that the case, that the fishy odor is from decomposition? It's because of a chemical called *trimethylamine*. Trimethylamine is the chemical compound responsible for both the well-known aroma of decomposing fish and for some abnormal vaginal odors from those annoying bad bacteria.

Earthy or BO type

There are two main types of sweat glands in our bodies. Sweat glands are responsible for helping to maintain body temperature and can also respond to stress. The first type of glands are called eccrine and are distributed throughout the body to help to cool you down. The other type of glands are the apocrine. These are found in your armpits and groin area. That earthy BO smell can be found in both those places. Some people's concentrations of these glands are higher than others, and that's why and how your personal odor changes and differs from other people. This is generally normal but may change with stress, weight, and diet.

Sweet

There are a couple of different kinds of sweet vaginal smell, one normal and one not quite so normal, and sometimes it's hard to tell the difference between the two. An overgrowth of yeast in the vagina can produce a sweet smell, somewhat similar to that of cookies or honey. Remember that yeast overgrowth is usually accompanied by some other symptoms like irritation or itching. Now, a sweet like molasses odor, just barely perceptible, is probably normal and is attributed to a normal shift in your healthy vaginal bacteria.

Chemical/Bleach

Semen has a high pH, and the seminal fluid may have a bleachy smell. So in the hours or day or so after sex you may detect a bleachy odor.

This will usually flush itself out over several days, so there is no need to urinate or douche after sex. Also, urine itself includes a substance called urea, which is a byproduct of ammonia. You may smell this odor more often if you are dehydrated.

Tangy

The pH of your healthy vagina is slightly acidic. This is what gives the vagina its baseline odor. In fact, it's quite common. Think about sourdough bread and some beers.

Metallic

That metallic smell you may notice is usually from blood at menstruation, because blood has iron in it. This smell may linger for a few days after your period. Sex can also cause a metallic odor due to the interaction of semen with vaginal fluid, which may temporarily alter your pH. It's rare that a metallic odor is a bigger problem.

Pheromones

These don't smell like anything, and there is some debate as to whether or not they actually exist. The data tells us no, so let's just leave it there.

Is my discharge normal?

Now that we've reviewed some of the smells that can come out of your vagina, let's talk about what types of discharge comes out of the vagina. General types of vaginal discharge considered normal and not normal are touched upon below. Keep in mind this is just a rule of thumb, and always see a practitioner if you're unsure.

Watery/clear: normal

If you drink a lot of water, your vagina will excrete watery discharge. Also, a small amount of discharge in your underwear is healthy. Think about how much saliva your body makes to keep your mouth moist. You don't notice it because you swallow it. Well, your vagina can't do that, so some must come out.

White, thick, and mucusy: normal

This happens mostly at midcycle, at ovulation. This mucus is produced to help sperm stick to the cervix and get inside the uterus for conception. It also looks like egg whites.

Yellow and thick: possibly abnormal

Could it be yeast? Drink some water, take off the thong, ditch the leggings, and wait a bit. You could simply be dehydrated. If it's still annoying you, see your doc. We want to rule out any sexually transmitted infection such as chlamydia or gonorrhea. If you are menopausal, this type of discharge may be due to a non-infectious condition called *atrophic vaginitis*, otherwise known as the *genitourinary syndrome* of menopause, and it is usually treated with vaginal estrogens.

Green: probably abnormal

If it's copious and accompanied by an abnormal odor, we think trichomonas. Yeast can also be greenish, but this discharge is usually thick and clumpy.

Blue: probably abnormal

Just checking to see if you're reading this. The only time you see blue discharge is in a maxi pad advertisement.

Brownish: possibly normal

If it's right after or just before your period, it's probably blood. Know that once blood hits the air, it becomes oxidized and changes color to a brownish hue over time. This may also happen at the middle of your cycle when you ovulate. If it's been a chunk of time since you've had a Pap and this happens after sex, your cervix may have an abnormality and you should have a Pap test. Cancer, unfortunately, is associated with bloody, mucusy discharge with a foul odor.

DID YOU KNOW?

Women have been associated with fish since ancient times. In Greek and Syrian cultures, the words for "fish" and "womb" are synonymous, and the Syrian goddess Atargatis was pictured as a mermaid. The well-known ichthys, or fish symbol, was once a pagan symbol for women and fertility. So much for that fishy smell . . .[2]

8

Why Do We Call It Pussy?

Call a thing what it is. Intimate is NOT my vagina.

—ME

When I was 5 years old, my mom took me to the pediatrician for some reason or another. While we were there, the doctor asked me if I needed to go pee-pee. I promptly responded, "I do not pee; I urinate." The doctor was so impressed with my early command of the English language (thanks, of course, to my teacher mother) that he was speechless. Using our incredible language properly has apparently been my modus operandi since the beginning. Of course we know that *pee-pee* is urinating, but do we always equate *pussy* with vagina? Likely so, but why the euphemism?

It is important for us to understand the words associated with our genitalia and brandish them as our armor and our pride. Throughout history, there seems to be a need to somehow mask, hide, or otherwise cloak the terms for genitalia of both genders. The terms for women, however, are much more disgusting, often overtly sexist, and far less humorous than those of our male counterparts. When I hear my patients reluctant to refer to their vaginas by the proper term and offer euphemisms for her, like *vajayjay*, I am dismayed that in this so-called modern era women are still afraid to call "the vajayjay" what it is, a vagina. *Va·gi·na*, pronounced *və-jī-nə*, from the Latin meaning "sword sheath"—an origin that oddly, but unsurprisingly, seems to have more to do with penises. Regardless, it is the most widely used term we have. When we ourselves don't refer to her in the proper terms we allow the vilification of our vaginas to become complete, and it's time for that to stop.

In order to take ownership of our vaginas, let us explore the words that we have chosen to represent her instead of her real name and the interesting origins of words like *pussy*. As a student of language, I am endlessly fascinated by how words develop and why and how we use them. Let us start with the ever-fascinating overuse of the word *intimate* on every maxi-pad-tampon-period-panty-vagina-deodorant-ad on earth.

STOP CALLING IT *INTIMATE*

The word *intimate* has nothing to do with your vagina. It's not even in the dictionary as being related to vaginas or female genitalia at all. Here is the etymology of the word (word origins being of utmost importance because they should guide their usage):

> **In·ti·mate**
> Pronounciation: \ ˈin(t)ə mət \
> *Adjective.* From the Latin word intimus which means,
> "inmost, innermost, deepest."

The word came into use in the 1630s. Intimate can also be taken as a noun, a "familiar friend, person with whom one is intimate." The word became associated with women's underwear around 1921. Soon thereafter, we got "intimate" everything. Looking up the term *intimate health* in a search engine will yield more than 210 million results. Why can't we use the word *vaginal* or *vulvar* health? Or even *penile* health, for that matter?

We are talking about the health of genitalia, right? The answer lies in advertising's desire to remain inoffensive, which makes for creative verbiage. You can't even put up an ad that uses the word *vagina* on most of the major social media sites. I've tried. Unfortunately, when we marginalize the proper term, we demonize it, causing us to use inappropriate words like *intimate* and making us all look like puritans.[1]

WHERE DID THE TERM *PUSSY* COME FROM?

A quick search of the Merriam-Webster Dictionary demonstrates several known and some lesser-known meanings of *pussy*. Note the pronunciations as well:

Pus·sy
Pronunciation: \ ˈpu̇-sē \
Plural: Pussies

Noun **1:** CAT **2:** a catkin of the pussy willow

Noun **1 vulgar:** VULVA **2 vulgar:** SEXUAL INTERCOURSE
2b vulgar: the female partner in sexual intercourse

Noun
Slang: A weak or cowardly man or boy: WIMP, SISSY

Adjective
Pronunciation: \ ˈpə-sē \
pussier; pussiest
Full of or resembling pus
a pussy wound

How many times have you actually used the word *pussy* to mean cat? It's uncommon in the US, but cats and vaginas have been intertwined for centuries, across cultures.

Perhaps one of the earliest uses of the word *puss* to mean anything female can be found in a book of folk songs from 1698. The songwriter describes the tendency of the day for men to marry early and to as young a girl as possible. "Honour" is taken as marriage in this case:

> *Honour's a Toy,*
>
> *For Fools a Decoy,*
>
> *Beset with Care and Fear;*
>
> *And that (I wuss)*
>
> *Kills many a Puss,*
>
> *Before her clymacht Year*

Clymacht is an old English word, equivalent to our modern English *climacteric*. In this song, the word *clymacht* could mean a critical or very important event, or flowering or ripening of fruit. When cast in this light, one may be inclined to believe that very young women are being wed off and die before menopause, a likely phenomenon in the late 1600s. However, the other meaning of *climacteric* is the onset of menopause, which is probably the true meaning, given childbirth was the most desired goal for marriage during those times. Of course, it's hard to know what the songwriter meant, or where he got that particular word to feature in the song, but this might be the earliest use of *puss* in relation to females. My best guess is that he really needed something to rhyme with *wuss*. Or maybe it was the other way around?

Another alleged origin of the word *pussy* came from a lewd country song from a similar time and place. Perhaps these songwriting men even knew each other. I can easily imagine these two old English gentlemen in a pub discussing their conquests over delicious, warm British beer, each exaggerating over the other about who got the best pussy. In the first stanza of this song (not reproduced here), Thomas D'Urfey imagines a young woman wed off to a much older man who has been left sexually unsatisfied. Read the song, and I'll add in some color commentary and translation as needed:[2]

A Pretty young Kitty,

She had that could Purr;

'Twas gamesome and handsome,

And had a rare Furr;

[remember they kept the hair down there,

so it was seen as sexy]

And straight up I took it, and offer'd to stroke it,

[cunnilingus]

In hopes I should make it kind;

But lowting and powting,

It still was to me,

Tho' Nature, the Creature,

Design'd should be free.

[the young girl wasn't attracted to her older

husband and wanted something else]

I play'd with its Whiskers and would have had discourse,

But ah! it was dumb and blind:

[not receptive to him at all]

When Cloris unquiet, who knew well its diet,

[Cloris = clitoris]

And found that I wanted that,

Cry'd pray, Run, fetch John,

[John was a well-known term for penis

at that time, like Johnson today]

He's the Man that can,

When it does need it, best know how to feed it,

Or gad you will starve my Cat.

[The next stanza features the actual word for pussy.

So exciting; here we go!]

As Fleet as my Feet

Could convey me I sped;

To Johnny who many

Times Pussey had fed.

[The boyfriend John, or at least John's penis,

had serviced this pussy in the past]

I told him my Errand, he wanted no warrant,

But hasted to shew his skill:

He took it to stroak it,

And close in his lap

He laid it to feed it,

And gave it some Pap;

And with such a passion it took the Collation,

Its belly began to fill,

[she became pregnant]

And now within Door is, so merry my Cloris,

She laughs and grows wonderous fat,

[allusion to pregnancy again]

And I run for John,

Who's the Man that can,

Tho' I'm at distance, give present assistance,

To please her, and feed her Cat.[3]

This poem clearly relates the word *pussy* to both cat and vagina, so it appears that England in the late 1600s is where the relationship between *cat* and *vagina* was solidified in the wider European culture, and vaginas and cats have walked hand in hand ever since. Remember the pink pussycat hats of the 2016 Women's March, when we said "pussy grabs back"? Now you know from whence it came, and pussy knowledge is pussy power!

Puss the cat and pussy the vagina established themselves in broader European culture in a close timeline. The French word for cat, *le chat*, is well-known to have a double meaning. In fact, a popular play called *L'Ecole des Femmes* (*School for Wives*) is a rather interesting story with the double entendre for *le chat* (cat/pussy, etc.). In this story, we find another older gentleman trying to control a younger woman. This gentleman, Arnolphe, conspires to keep his young female charge completely unaware of the perils and pleasures of the world. Unfortunately for him, he leaves his young, attractive male protegé in charge of her for an extended length of time. In one scene, Agnes, the young girl, freely admits to Arnolphe losing a particularly treasured cat-like object to the dashing young man. Please forgive my translation from the French:

> **Arnolphe:** *What's new?*
>
> **Agnes:** *My little cat is dead.*
>
> **Arnolphe:** *Too bad; but what (can we do)!*
> *We are all mortal, and each of us will.*
>
> The scene progresses to a point where Arnolphe thinks aloud
> (in a Shakespearean way)
>
> **Arnolphe:** *The world, dear Agnes, is a strange thing!*
> *See how everyone backbites!*
> *Some neighbors told me that a young man*
> *Was, in my absence, at home;*
> *That you had suffered his sight and his harangues.*
> *But I have not taken faith in these wicked languages,*
> *And I wanted to bet that it was false.*
>
> **Agnes:** *Don't bet! You'd surely lose . . . .*

"My little cat is dead" (*Le petit chat est mort*) = (loose translation) losing virginity.

French cats and French vaginas seem to be quite familiar with one another, *n'est-ce pas?* The French give us another play on the vagina and the cat: The 19th-century French nightclub Le Chat Noir, The Black Cat, was one of the first cabarets and featured female entertainment similar to that of the more well-known Moulin Rouge.

FIG. 8.1

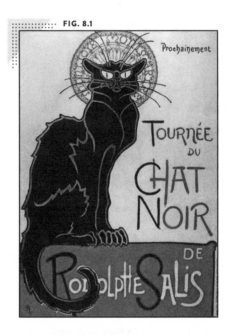

THE 1896 POSTER ADVERTISING THE BLACK CAT CLUB "COMING SOON."

Soft, pleasant things such as kitty cats and furry vaginas have had a universal appeal throughout time and culture, which may be why the two are forever intertwined. Early America also has its mentions of the term *pussy*. However, unlike the uses in England or France, *pussy* in this country was used to refer to children, primarily little girls. For example, take the 1852 novel *Uncle Tom's Cabin* by Harriet Beecher Stowe. During a conversation in which the very nature of slavery is defended (that requires a whole other book to discuss), Augustine St. Clare, one of Uncle Tom's owners, converses with another character. *Pussy* appears to be a normal term of endearment used for his little daughter, Eva:

*"Well, at any rate," said Marie, as she reclined herself on a
lounge, "I'm thankful I'm born where slavery exists; and I
believe it's right,—indeed, I feel it must be; and, at any rate,
I'm sure I couldn't get along without it."*

*"I say, what do you think, Pussy?" said her father to Eva,
who came in at this moment, with a flower in her hand.*

"What about, papa?"

*"Why, which do you like the best—to live as they do
at your uncle's, up in Vermont, or to have a house-full of
servants, as we do?"*

"O, of course, our way is the pleasantest," said Eva.

"Why so?" said St. Clare, stroking her head.

*"Why, it makes so many more round you to love, you
know," said Eva, looking up earnestly.*

*"Now, that's just like Eva," said Marie; "just one of her
odd speeches."*

*"Is it an odd speech, papa?" said Eva, whisperingly, as she
got upon his knee.*

"Rather, as this world goes, Pussy," said St. Clare.[4]

And thus, we have one of the earliest well-known American uses of the word *pussy*, having nothing to do with a vagina and forever associated with a book on the defense of slavery.

Not to be outdone by England and France and even the United States, there are a few other contenders for the mantle of the origin of *pussy*. Both the Nordic and German languages use a similar word. The Old Norse word *puss* means "pocket or pouch" and Low German's *puse* means "vulva." Consider how small Europe is. As people move about from country to country, their words often follow and end up blending together, either with the same or multiple meanings, so it stands to reason that these terms found their ways in and out of various languages and cultures throughout history and time. Vaginas as pockets have even found their way into modern-day use. Consider this 21st-century quotation:

"The vah-yine-yah is nature's pocket.
It's natural, and it's responsible."
—Ilana Glazer from Comedy Central's *Broad City*

Pussy-whipped is another term derived from the *p* word. As you may know, it is used to indicate a man who has been rendered submissive to his mate's vagina. The origin of *pussy-whipped* dates back to the late 1950s and portrays a man subservient to his woman, subject to her whims and desires because of his access (or lack thereof) to sex. *Pussy-whipped* seems to have first appeared in 1956 (its 15th-century Middle English predecessor is *cunt-beaten*, meaning "impotent"). However, my favorite version is the German *unter dem Pantoffel*, which is literally translated as "under the slipper," as in a women's shoe.[5]

We must harken back to traditional gender roles to understand why *pussy-whipped* exists in the first place. No one ever said a woman was *penis-whipped*, and if they did, they were probably referring to domestic violence. We must consider what has become the derogatory nature of *pussy*, progressing from benign and sweet as referred to in *Uncle Tom's Cabin* to vicious and sinister. It connotes a self-perceived loss of control of the male in a male/female relationship. Of course, when the woman has an equal say, then the man *must* be "whipped." If a man picks up the phone immediately when his girlfriend/significant other/spouse calls, or heads right over when she asks, he *must* be whipped. If a man washes a dish while the woman works, oh he is *certainly* whipped. It is these misconstrued notions of male dominance that have existed since antiquity that we must work to overcome for any type of gender equity to truly exist. Then there will be no need for anyone to be pussy-whipped.

CUNT . . . THERE, I SAID IT

It would seem that from the beginning the use of the word *cunt* has been extraordinarily derogatory. But we are intrepid explorers of the pussydom in all its forms and likenesses, and thus we dive in and discover what knowledge can be found.[6] And what we will learn is that there is more to *cunt* than meets the eye.

Cunt has its share of origin stories just like your "intimate pussy." It appears that its first modern appearance was, again, in Olde England. Around 1230, a certain street known to be the place for sex workers was called, seriously, Gropecunte Lane. As the story goes, London's street names evolved basically from whatever happened nearby. By 1310, prostitution was officially restricted to outside the city of London. However, there are several instances of Gropecunt, Gropekunte, and Gropecunte Lanes popping up all around London. Given the notoriously difficult-to-navigate streets of London, this name was not only descriptive but useful for those traveling businessmen who would know exactly where to go to find what they were looking for.[7]

We can also look to the ancient East. There is a certain Hindu goddess whose name is Kunti. When translated, it means the "Yoni of the Universe." Nice, right? Truth be told, *cunt*, with its relationship to goddesses, has a more feminist origin than *vagina*. The Yoni Cunt-Goddess represented the power and beauty of the female body in its glorious strength. Taken from the *Mahabharata*, an ancient historical Hindu text from sometime between 200 and 400 BCE, Kunti led a matriarchy that rivaled many male-led family lines. In fact, *cunt* is related to words from China, Rome, Ireland, Egypt, and I'm quite sure many others. In contrast to the derogatory sense of the word in our "modern society," it was simply a matter-of-fact and respectful title for priestesses, witches, and women in general.

> *In ancient writings, the word for "cunt" was synonymous with "woman," though not in the insulting sense. An Egyptologist was shocked to find the maxims of Ptah-Hotep "used for 'woman' a term that was more than bling," though its indelicacy was not in the eye of the ancient beholder, only in that of the modern one.*[8]

The word *cunt* as a derogatory term appears to have been enshrined by the 1920s. But why? Why did this one single-syllable word come to have such a heinous meaning that it is barely uttered in polite society? Imagine this word in your mind. *CUNT*. It bites when you speak it. The fact that it is monosyllabic gives it punch, like *fuck*. Perhaps these two words walk hand in hand, historically speaking. Maybe *cunt* holds such power because it starts with that hard C sound. Form a C with your mouth. It comes from a place in the back of the throat, almost as if you have to dig deeply to form it.

Why are we so afraid of *cunt*? I think the answer is simple: While there are very few truly derogatory words for male anatomy that insinuate lack of cleanliness and perpetuate disgust, we have plenty for women, and for some reason, *cunt* has evolved in our language as the most disgusting. I say we take back our cunts and all the words that stand in for our vaginas and recognize the fear and power inherent in our bodies—pussy, cunt, vagina, and all!

Ethel Merman was a well-known Broadway actress known for playing "broads" in the 1930s. Born in 1908, she made her name in such now-classic musicals as *Hello Dolly*, *Annie Get Your Gun*, and *Anything Goes*. A comic at heart, she used her powerful voice on stage and screen to play many of musical comedy's quintessential leading ladies. Why am I telling you this? Well, there is a story about Ms. Merman, then in her fifties, coming back from filming a movie one day and announcing to her then-husband, Ernest Borgnine:

> *"The director said I looked sensational. He said I had the voice of a 20-year-old, the face of a 30-year-old, and the body and legs of a 35-year-old!"*
>
> *Borgnine replied: "Did he say anything about your 65-year-old cunt?"*
>
> *Merman replied: "No, he didn't mention you at all."*[9]

DID YOU KNOW?

The pussy hat was invented by Jayna Zweiman and Krista Suh in 2016 in response to the 45th U.S. president's 2005 comment that women would let him "grab them by the pussy." The hand-knitted hats, pink and shaped like pussycat ears, sparked a global protest movement, spawning the hashtag "#PussyGrabsBack" on Twitter.

9

Orgasming Vaginas

Good sex is like good bridge.
If you don't have a good partner,
you'd better have a good hand.

—MAE WEST

I s anyone else bothered by the fact that whenever someone writes about having an orgasm, they refer to it as *achieving orgasm*? I *achieved* obtaining a medical degree. I *have* orgasms.

Look at the cover of any women's magazine on any given month, and you will probably find something about the ever-elusive vaginal orgasm or some sex trick that will make you a powerhouse in bed and make him want to get down on his knees and propose immediately. You'll also find a thousand internet articles on achieving multiple female orgasms. You would think all American women are doing is walking around having orgasms. The mantra that sex sells rings true for women as well as men, just in a different way.

THE ORGASM GAP

Unfortunately, I often have patients who tell me they have never had an orgasm. This happens at least once a week, and at least one woman a day tells me she has problems with sex. And if I had a dollar for every patient who tells me she's never had an orgasm through penetrative sex, I could do my job for free. I'm here to tell you that has to change, because the orgasm gap is real.

It is estimated that up to 40 percent (yes, you read that right) of adult women of all sexual orientations report some type of sexual concern. This survey included women between the ages of 40 and 80. Younger women, however, are not immune.[1] Another study that surveyed about 800 college students of all genders found that only 39 percent of women said that they usually or always experienced orgasm in partnered (male-female) sex, compared to 91 percent of men—an "orgasm gap" of 52 percent.[2] Now, this is a book about vaginas, and partnered sex doesn't have to be the only way your vagina (we're talking about everything there, the clitoris especially) can experience pleasure. Unfortunately, there has been an overemphasis on sex as being solely a male-female activity. This is far from the case, and it is imperative that we discuss and celebrate vaginal pleasure in all its glorious forms.

Female pleasure has historically been misunderstood and mischaracterized, but it seems to be enjoying a sort of renaissance recently, with various products for sale all claiming to make you have an orgasm and make your orgasm better, such as the now infamous yoni egg. But in reality, no money needs to be spent to experience our innate sexual gifts, and those gifts are many, as women's capacity for orgasm is at least twice that of men. Comparatively speaking, women have twice as many nerve endings in the erogenous zones as men. The thinking that (cis) women experience greater sexual pleasure than men has been pervasive from the beginning, and therefore there may be some truth to the matter. And after reading this chapter, it is my hope that you will come to understand both the truth and the fallacy of this argument.

FEMALE PLEASURE IN HISTORY AND MYTHOLOGY

In ancient Greek mythology, there was a blind soothsayer called Tiresias. As one legend goes, Tiresias, who was able to move between the worlds of mortals and gods, accidentally stepped upon two snakes engaged in a rapturous embrace. Because snakes are the beloved animal of the goddess Hera (Zeus's consort) she punished (punished?) Tiresias by turning him into a woman for seven years. During his time as a female, he engaged in sex and even gave birth. This gives the character quite a unique perspective into intercourse from the perspective of both genders. The story goes that one day, Zeus and Hera, the god and goddess at the top of the chain, were having an argument over who experienced more pleasure during sex. To answer their question, they summoned Tiresias, given his experiences being male and female. His answer to the query was, of course, the female.

Female sexual pleasure is documented and featured prominently in many ancient cultures, but perhaps not more so than ancient India. Sexual pleasure overall, and female pleasure specifically, was emphasized here more than in most other ancient cultures, as famously documented in the *Kama Sutra*. A *sutra* is simply defined as a treatise. *Kama* is from the Sanskrit for "the enjoyment of appropriate objects by the five senses of hearing, feeling, seeing, tasting, and smelling, assisted by the mind together with the soul." Therefore, you can think of the document as a "Treatise on All Pleasure."

Written and compiled by Vatsyayana, the *Kama Sutra* is not simply a book of sex positions, as is widely thought. It has sections on society and hierarchy, attraction, and even infidelity, appearing to emphasize religious duty, wealth, and status, as well as carnal pleasure, as part of a greater continuum. In the very first chapter of the *Kama Sutra*, the writer states that pleasure is an essential part of life: "Pleasures, being as necessary for the existence and well-being of the body as food . . ." Part one of the *Kama Sutra* discusses mankind and its role in obtaining religious enlightenment, study, and the gaining of wealth and friends all as being part of pleasure. But, of course, the most popular part of the text is the part about intercourse, and in it female pleasure is focused upon specifically.

History professor Anne Hardgrove writes in the introduction to a newly released version of the *Kama Sutra* a most interesting observation: "Significantly, the *Kama Sutra* provided a major contribution to sexual knowledge because of its emphasis on female pleasure. According to the *Kama Sutra*, for a marriage to be successful, happy, and stable, it is the man's responsibility and duty that his wife should derive pleasure from sex."[3] Insofar as the female orgasm can be described, the *Kama Sutra* doesn't do such a bad job. It instructs the male partner in foreplay, congress, and even what to do after sex is over. The book describes the female orgasm as a sign of "enjoyment and satisfaction" when she literally "puts aside all bashfulness" and "brings the two organs together," and it encourages the partner to use fingers to stroke and rub to ensure pleasure has taken place. The *Kama Sutra* also advises that the woman should climax first and discusses the concept of multiple orgasms. Compared to men, the *Kama Sutra* admits that it is "impossible" for a woman to describe her pleasure, and goes on to explain that the male partner, once he "emits" is essentially satisfied, but also states that this is "not so with the females." It seems to insinuate that either further pleasure is possible, or that men are completely unaware as to whether or not the female in a male-female partnership has had at least one orgasm.

Now, let's look at another 15th-century ancient Indian text. This one, written by the Hindu poet Kalyanamally, was commissioned by a Muslim ruler, Ladakhana. It promotes fidelity by advising couples to bring variety to the marriage bed. What is most fascinating about this text is that it is so specific on parts of women's bodies and what can result in sexual arousal. The text refers to women as "centers of passion" and involves many parts of the body that one may not think of as erogenous—but hey, it may be worth a try! For example, they recommend pressing the knee, pressing the foot with a toe, and pressing the calf muscle. While that may be useful after a run, I'm not sure if it is particularly erogenous. However, they may be on to something, given that the text is thousands of years old. Perhaps it can't hurt to nibble on a knee?

Rome also had some understanding of the importance of pleasure, and despite their general obsession with documentation of legality and Catholic canon law, there were a few Romans who produced some enlightened thoughts about sex. Of course, it was believed that the primary reason for copulation was reproduction, but there were some who believed that reproduction required orgasms from both parties. Take Paolo Zacchia, for example. In the 1600s, he was basically the Surgeon General of Rome. Going against the popular thought of the day and disagreeing even with the likes of Aristotle, who had asserted that "seed" was only produced by the male, Zacchia wrote that in order for full coitus to exist, women also had to produce "seed." This was not a prelude to the knowledge of sperm and egg, but rather it implied that the wife should "also experience pleasure from coitus." He wrote that "the husband who does not make room for his wife's pleasure is likely to fail double since her pleasure is necessary to produce the seed, which will be needed for generation." It's almost too bad that this has been proven wrong.[4]

THE NECTAR OF THE GODS

Ernst Gräfenberg (1881–1957) was a German gynecologist who accomplished many things during his career. He came up with theories on how cancer metastasizes, developed an IUD, and studied the anatomy of the female urethra. This is where things get interesting and how his name lives in infamy—it is after him that the G-spot is named. Dr Gräfenberg wrote about what would later become known as the G-spot in 1950, describing the nerves around the urethral sphincter and anterior part of the vagina where the spot is thought to be located. It was described as a sensitive area that can be detected through the front vaginal wall, which swells when manipulated in a certain fashion. This has led some to believe that the

G-spot may be a source of the ever-elusive vaginal orgasm and perhaps even female ejaculation.

The vaginal orgasm and female ejaculation are controversial subjects, but evidence of these phenomena in relation to the G-spot have been around for a very long time. Ancient cultures worldwide have observed and reported a certain aspect of urethral activity during intercourse as an indication of pleasure.

In ancient India, China, and Greece, medical scholarly writers observed and documented this phenomenon. Aristotle documented the emission of a female fluid around 300 BCE, as did Galen in the 2nd century CE. The Romans called these fluids "liquor vitae," vital fluid. In Chinese Tao-ist texts from the 4th century, there is mention of female ejaculation. In India, the 3rd-century *Kama Sutra* does not mention female ejaculation. However, by the 11th and 13th centuries, texts like the *Pancasayaka* and *Jayamangala*, written as commentary and expansion on the *Kama Sutra*, document the existence of the G-spot and female ejaculation in great detail. They called this fluid *amrita*, or "nectar of the gods."[5]

Female ejaculation refers to about a teaspoon's worth of fluid expelled through the urethra that looks like watered-down fat-free milk. Science has actually examined this fluid and determined that it is chemically similar to fluid found in the male prostate called *prostate-specific antigen*. It also contains glucose and fructose (a type of sugar). So there must be a reason that this fluid was called "nectar," right? Some ancient explorer had to have had a taste.

In 1981, while doing research into Kegel muscle exercises for urinary incontinence, a team of medical doctors and nurse practitioners made an interesting discovery. They examined over four hundred women and found a sensitive area that swells when it is stimulated with a "come hither" motion, in all the women they studied. This phenomenon appeared to them to mirror Dr. Gräfenburg's description circa 1950, and they named it after him, the G-spot. They also found that ejaculation is variable, and that some women ejaculate with or even without orgasm, or have orgasm without ejaculating.[6]

In Dr. Gräfenburg's words, "Analogous to the male urethra, the female urethra also seems to be surrounded by erectile tissues like the corpora cavernosa." This means that similar to a penile erection indicating desire for sex, the tissue right over the vagina has this function as well.[7]

Despite two thousand years of documentation, many academics fail to acknowledge that it is possible for a woman to experience pleasure vaginally. Academics call the evidence for vaginal pleasure and even orgasm "anecdotal" and "flimsy." In fact, you can still google the deniers. Even the *Huffington Post* called the concept of the G-spot "a myth." I am going to go out on a limb and argue that there may not be a "spot" per se, but there is certainly enough data and anatomical observations demonstrating that the tissues in the anterior (front) portion of the vagina are part of the extension of the clitoris, now known as the bulb or root.[8]

Although there is plenty of controversy surrounding the G-spot, the data we have appears to be on Dr. Gräfenburg's side, and it is growing. In 1990, an anonymous questionnaire was reported in the *Archives of Sexual Behavior*.[9] This questionnaire was distributed to 2,350 professional women in the United States and Canada. About 55 percent of the women returned the survey. Of these women, 40 percent reported having a fluid release (ejaculation) at the moment of orgasm. In addition, 82 percent of the women who reported having the sensitive area (good old Dr. Gräfenberg's spot) also reported ejaculation with their orgasms. These women described that the orgasm felt deeper inside their body and felt like a "bearing down" sensation, like the uterus is pushing into the vagina. And there even is more research from doctors who do nothing but study anatomy that shows the connection between pleasure and this particular part of the vagina. As late as 2017, there were still papers being published about this pleasurable area that we know *has to exist*. These papers appear to walk a fine line, acknowledging that this part of the vagina is the "most sensitive," but not calling it the G-spot specifically.[10] As far as I am concerned, who cares what you call it—we know it exists.

EMBRACING THE ORGASM

It is exactly because of this denial of female pleasure that women still have the problem of being at home with our sexuality and the nature of our pleasure. Despite historical documentation from these most fascinating texts and new anatomical knowledge that brings us into the 20th and 21st centuries, female sexual pleasure as a right has yet to be fully embraced by society as a whole. This is why certain magazines and associated websites still talk about it as if it's some brand-new thing to discover.

Since the United States were founded by Puritans, can we expect much in the promotion of a sexually educated and liberated society? All too often women focus their pleasure not on themselves, but on their partners. This is why lesbian partners are documented as reporting more orgasms; each partner is probably placing value on the other one's pleasure. We as women place ourselves second all the time in work and family life, and unfortunately that doesn't appear to stop at the bedroom. Again, this harkens back to the founding of our nation on Puritanical mores and the roles that gender plays in society, despite how far we have come in attempting to achieve some semblance of equanimity or at least parity.

This suppression of such a vital part of human nature, the meaningful pursuit of pleasure, has resulted in a massive underground market for myriad ways to release repressed sexual tension, and likely manifests itself in various anxieties and quite possibly depression. This tension, bred from the bevy of misinformation that has permeated society, results in women who are genuinely afraid to embrace their own sexual power, their sexuality, and their natural ability to experience pleasure. They are often afraid of sex itself, and the reasons are probably quite complex.

Consider the status of the relationship between partners, the presence or absence of children, and other life stressors. All these in various combinations can contribute to sexual difficulty. In my practice, a majority of my patients with sexual pain and lack of orgasm suffer also from anxiety, depression, or both. Given the fact that there are twice as many nerves in the clitoris (approximately eight thousand) as in the glans penis or the tip (approximately four thousand), why is there still an orgasm gap in heterosexual sex? The medical community has attempted to give some relief, but the pursuit is far from complete.

Part of that effort is to offer a few known medical treatments to aid in improving sexual function and create better orgasming vaginas. Keep in mind, all this info is just for you to know your options; it's not medical advice for you specifically. Make sure to talk to your own physician or practitioner to explore what may be right for *you*.

Female Viagra

In 2015, a so-called "female Viagra" was brought to market. With the scientific name flibanserin, this pill was meant to treat a woman's lack of desire. It is a little pink pill, compared to Viagra's little blue one. However, it differs in function from Viagra (sildenafil), which helps a man who already has the desire for sex achieve the physical male necessity for sex, an erection, by redirecting blood flow. The female version works by acting on the brain to increase certain neurotransmitters, mainly dopamine and norepinephrine. It also decreases another neurotransmitter, serotonin. We know that dopamine is an important part of the reward (pleasure) system in the brain, and increasing dopamine even a small amount is enough to send lab rats into a tizzy. The release of large amounts of this neurotransmitter are what makes certain street drugs so addictive. It's also one of the things that happen when you have an orgasm.

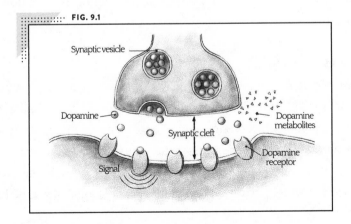

FIG. 9.1

HOW NEUROTRANSMITTERS WORK IN THE BRAIN.

Pleasurable and excitatory activity is driven by dopamine and norepinephrine, and inhibitory activity is driven by serotonin. Keeping these neurotransmitter systems in balance is important to achieve a normal sexual response. According to the study for this drug's approval, this medication increased "satisfying sexual events" from 2.7 to 3.7 per month.[11] This is a modest improvement at best, likely proving to us that sexual function depends on much more than neurotransmitters. Unfortunately, the biggest side effect with this medication is sedation, which is sort of like slipping yourself a mickey.

Self-injections

Another treatment new to the market, which also works on neurotransmitters, is bremelanotide, trade name Vyleesi, which activates multiple alternative receptors in the brain besides dopamine. The knowledge of different receptors affecting sexual function shows us that this whole orgasm and pleasure thing is quite the complex process, and there may not be one shot to cure all. This medication is given by a tiny injection similar to that used for diabetes, in a fleshy part of the body, like the thigh. According to the drug's qualifying study, the improvement in sexual function is moderate, with about 25 percent of the patients demonstrating an increase in satisfaction, and 35 percent of patients reporting a decrease in dissatisfaction.[12] If your sexual function is so compromised that a small improvement will suffice, it may be worth considering as an option with your practitioner.

Viagra (sildenafil)

The use of actual Viagra by women has also been documented, with hit-or-miss results just like the other drugs. It appears to have a similar effect in women as in men, increasing genital engorgement. In one study some women with a diagnosis of depression did get a boost in sexual arousal and orgasm, but the study only looked at about a hundred women. Another study, which involved nearly eight hundred women, found it was no better than a sugar pill.[13] So despite the fact that, physiologically, Viagra accomplishes a similar effect, sexual arousal itself is more than just blood flow, especially for us vagina owners.

Platelet-rich plasma injection

(They call this the Oh-Shot. I can't use the actual name because it's trademarked.) Platelet-rich plasma, PRP for short, is a type of injection purported to improve orgasm. It involves the use of your own blood serum, which contains growth factors, or your platelet-rich plasma. Injected into the area in and around the clitoris, it is said to improve the clitoris's responsiveness to stimulation. Blood serum does contain multiple scientifically proven growth factors. In fact, it's been used to treat other areas of the body: arthritic knees, back pain and injury, and even male pattern baldness with varying results and mostly positive studies. The single study in support of female orgasm enhancement that is cited most often involved only eleven women, which is not a lot.[14] What this tells me again is that women's sexual health has been largely ignored by the scientific community as fringe. Unfortunately, this leaves me as a physician and you as a patient without much definitive knowledge, so the decision to partake in this treatment might be fraught with uncertainty.

Laser vaginal treatments

Laser vaginal treatment involves the use of laser light to heat the top layers of the vaginal tissue, causing the lower layers to make more collagen. Of all of the vaginal treatments, CO_2 lasers have the most information to back them up, because they have been in existence since the early 2000s. The first one was called the Mona Lisa Touch. And before you roll your eyes at the name, know that I rolled mine first. Comparing their laser to a great work of art is a bit of a stretch, no? Either way, nearly 50 percent of menopausal women complain of vaginal dryness, itching, and burning at some time in their lives. Studies suggest that the laser treatment is as effective and safe as vaginal estrogen in improving sexual and urinary functionality, meaning you can use this and not have to worry about creams or suppositories.[15]

This treatment may also be good for breast cancer survivors who are not able to use estrogen for their vaginal issues. Results of the VeLVET (Vaginal Laser Therapy to Vaginal Estrogen Therapy) trial have been published in the journal *Menopause*, the journal of the North American Menopause Society (NAMS).

Now you might say, "Hey, I'm not menopausal. Can this do anything for me?" When it comes to the big O, we don't have a lot of data except on menopausal women, and they did say it improved their sexual function, so take away what you will. There is one thing we do have actual information about: If you have a little leak when you cough, sneeze, or run, there is some good evidence this may help you out. The main problem I see with laser therapy is the cost. This is how corporations keep women from getting access to the technology that could really help them.

Think about this: The costs for technology like CT and MRI keep decreasing, but the cost for laser therapy is still in the thousands, despite the fact that lasers keep getting less and less expensive to make. So unfortunately, your doctor has to buy a laser for around $150K from the company that makes them. That company sees a hefty profit, and the doctors are left to try to recuperate the costs and pass that burden on to you. I have firsthand knowledge of this.[16]

Radiofrequency

This treatment is a single thirty-minute session where a little wand is rubbed across all the sections of the vagina. Imagine trying to lie back and relax for thirty minutes while someone is moving a little wand in, out, and around your vagina. (Pause. Awkward, right?) The study of premenopausal women I found says that 43.5 percent of women reported no more vaginal laxity and also registered an improvement in sexual function. It might work, and the studies seem to say it does help with laxity, but the thought of thirty minutes of this is just too much for even me to handle.[17]

Extracorporeal sound/shock wave therapy

There are more than thirty studies detailing various levels of use and effectiveness of sound wave therapy to treat erectile dysfunction and lots of anecdotal evidence. One person claimed in a blog post that it increased his masturbation frequency 1–2 times per day and that his "animal instinct" was "more intense."[18] However, I have not been able to find a single study about sound/shock wave therapy and the female orgasm although, in theory, the treatment shows promise.

Think about it like this: The central tenet of medicine is do no harm. As long as things are not worsened, and your condition could quite possibly improve, use your best judgment. It might be worth a go. All sorts of tech for men have been adapted for women, and only time and study will tell us how effective they really are.

Cognitive behavioral therapies

Because orgasm is a multifactorial process, let us also examine some of the psychological interventions in academic medicine. These are called cognitive behavioral therapies. Most of these therapies evolved during the sexual revolution of the 1960s and the women's liberation movement of the 1970s and are still in use today. We will discuss these a bit more when we discuss "Vaginas in Peril" in chapter 10, but for pleasure purposes, there is one particular therapy that stands out to me: sensate focus exercises.

This is a partnered exercise, usually directed by a therapist, that begins with prolonged eye contact and touch of non-erogenous zones and progresses to actual sex. With each therapy session—some sessions are done directly with a therapist and others are done at home—you progress over time to touching breasts, buttocks, and then genitals, in a certain fashion. The exercise focuses on pleasurable touch rather than orgasm as an endpoint. Sessions can last up to an hour each and are performed over several months' time. This particular therapy is also a type of desensitization therapy. The idea is not to desensitize you to sex, but to desensitize you to the stressors and anxiety surrounding it. Academic studies have shown an increase in the level of enjoyment of sexual caressing and in partnered intercourse frequency. Orgasmic responsiveness, however, was not affected. If you think about it, though, these were short-term studies, and because we know that the O is multifactorial, over time I would bet that the orgasming vagina would come around, literally.[19]

This is how sensate focus goes:[20]

You start with a commitment. This is going to take a while. You'll need to set aside at least one hour two or three times a week for you and your partner. Disconnect from any devices; you don't want to be distracted by social media or notifications. No alcohol, marijuana, drugs, or other mood-altering substances can be taken. This is something to focus on and savor, like a delicious meal.

Remove as much clothing as you feel comfortable. Nudity is best, but if you don't feel comfortable right away, start in robes or pajamas. You will also need some lighting so you can see each other's eyes and reactions. Proceed with these steps:

1. Take turns touching each other, but no sex and no touching nipples or genitals for the first several sessions. Also, use only nonverbal communication. For example, if you don't like where your partner is touching you at that particular moment, then gently guide their hand away. Remember, this is only to heighten sensitivity and awareness, so no kissing either, at least not at first. Use only hands, fingers, and limbs.

2. After you've mastered touching one another, then enjoy mutual touching. Still no kissing and no genital touching quite yet. Do this for another several sessions. There are five stages to the exercise. You're allowed to move to the next step after a few weeks of each.

3. After mutual touching has been done a few sessions, then it's OK to do a little exploration of the breasts and genitals. Keep in mind that this is not the main focus; you should simply add this touch to the other touch exercises.

4. Once you are comfortable with breast and genital exploration, then straddle your partner and allow your genitals to touch, but no insertion if male-female or male-male. Fingers are OK, though. You're almost there! It is important to take pains to ensure that each partner is comfortable with this step before you go to the last step.

5. The final step is genital insertion. This should be done very slowly, usually with female superior position. This will allow for greater control of insertion. Yahoo!

As long as no harm is done to your body, cognitive behavioral therapies may be a possible consideration, but keep in mind that the data, the real, hard data, is lacking for many of these. In addition, the supportive data we do have is either from small studies or only show a minimum of improvement. I've had patients who have had these treatments whose results reflect both sides of the spectrum. Some do incredibly well and experience a massive improvement, but a handful of others experience no benefit whatsoever. This tells us that more studies are needed to be able to prove yay or nay.

Also, consider the influence the mind has over the body, and in particular on the orgasm. If you are in touch with your body and have a positive mind-body relationship, you are probably more likely to benefit from these treatments. If your overall outlook on sexuality and the self has been obscured by outside factors such as a repressive upbringing or sexual trauma, there may be no pill, shot, suction cup, or anything that will make an orgasm happen for you. If that is the case, it may be time to explore other options to get back in touch with yourself and find your own orgasm in a different way.

Aphrodisiacs

There are herbal formulas or "aphrodisiacs" that can possibly help put us in the mood. Even the *Kama Sutra* talks about advising a woman to take "medicine to cause her desires to be satisfied quickly." Of course, what this mystery medicine may be is lost to history, but history also has been littered with various methods of inducing desire, and hopefully (though not necessarily) several orgasms. However, if we think of sexual satisfaction as a continuum from desire to orgasm and beyond, then we should at least touch on the subject.

Check out a few of the known aphrodisiacs throughout history:[21]

- Lilies: 3000 BCE, ancient Egypt
- The suckerfish/remora: 800 BCE, ancient Rome
- Cobra: 200 BCE, China
- Sea cucumber: 300 CE, China
- Saffron: 700 CE, Egypt and Greece
- Leafcutter ants: 1300 CE, Columbia
- Walnuts: 1400 CE, Switzerland
- Rhinoceros horn: 1600 CE, China
- Oysters: 1800 CE, Venice
  (The story goes that Casanova consumed these daily.)
- Blowfish: 1900 CE, Japan
- Tiger penis: 1900 CE, Southeast Asia
- Seahorses in alcohol: 1900 CE, China

FIG. 9.2

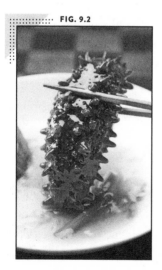

THE SEA CUCUMBER (SEEN HERE) IS THOUGHT TO BE AN APHRODISIAC.

Ambergris

Ambergris—a very distinct, naturally occurring material—has an earthy, woodsy, deep aroma that is wondrous, and as rumor has it, it's a highly effective aphrodisiac. It emanates from the belly of a whale who has tried to digest too many squid beaks and dies because of the obstruction. After the whale suffers from the obstruction, the rest of it is eaten away by sharks and other sea creatures. What's left is the beginning of ambergris.

The mass floats on the ocean and changes over time, from a dark waxy ball to a light grey, pumice stone–like material. An article in the *New York Times* from 1895 titled "Ambergris, the Whale Fisher's Prize," described its odor as being "like the blending of new–mown hay, the damp woodsy fragrance of a fern–copse, and the faintest possible perfume of the violet." They actually studied sexual responsiveness to ambergris, at least in male rats. The researchers found that male rats experienced—and this must be quoted to be believed—"recurrent episodes of penile erection, a dose-dependent, vigorous and repetitive increase in intromissions and an increased anogenital investigatory behavior." In non-absurd science-speak, the rats had more sex, both hetero- and homosexual, so it seems like there may be something to this, at least in rats. Nowadays, there is a synthetic version of ambergris available, so one doesn't have to wait on whale parts. Although not quite as amazing as the real thing, you can catch a whiff of it in some Chanel, Gucci, and Givenchy perfumes. Knowing where these perfumes come from gives you an entirely new perspective on things, doesn't it?[22]

Food and orgasms

In his book *Immoral Recipes*, the late Manuel Vázquez Montalbán writes, "No one has ever succeeded at seduction by means of food alone but there's a long list of those who have been seduced by talking about that which was to be eaten."[23] I certainly believe this to be true. M&M's or grocery store ramen noodles can be aphrodisiacs if delivered by the person you're hot for, or if you're just feeling yourself, so eat and enjoy.

Foodie-rumored aphrodisiacs include the following:[24]

- Sweets and spices: chocolate, sandalwood, tarragon, cinnamon, rosemary, lavender, garlic, ginger, vanilla, ginkgo, ginseng, mint, mustard, and chili pepper

- Miscellaneous proteins: bacon, cheese, eggs, nuts, and turkey
- Seafood: abalone, clams, blowfish, caviar, conch, sea urchin (uni), salmon, lobster, shrimp, sushi, tuna, mussels, sea cucumber, and, perhaps most famously, oysters
- Produce: truffle, avocado, arugula (rocket), basil, cucumber, pepper, tomato, pomegranate, celery, fennel, figs, mushrooms, asparagus, and seaweed

WHAT HAPPENS WHEN WE HAVE AN ORGASM?

Now, when we actually get to the part when we have an orgasm, what happens physically?

- Increase in heart rate
- Elevated blood pressure
- Increased levels of prolactin and oxytocin: Oxytocin is also fundamental in the labor and birthing process. This is why nipple stimulation and orgasm help to cause contractions and may also result in some cramping at orgasm.
- Nipple erection
- Congestion or swelling of the genitalia; you may feel your clitoris or vagina literally "beat" like your heart
- Muscle spasm

Masters and Johnson are the original, modern, self-purported sexual experts. They pioneered research on normal sexual function and were also of the belief that all orgasms essentially emanate from the clitoris. Their model of a five-step sexual response process has become the standard that we use today. They described what a vagina looks like at orgasm: The vagina balloons out and the uterus pulls up in response to clitoral stimulation. They were also the first modern researchers to publish observations of the multi-orgasmic female. Here's an overview on how anatomy and physiology play into normal sexual function.[25]

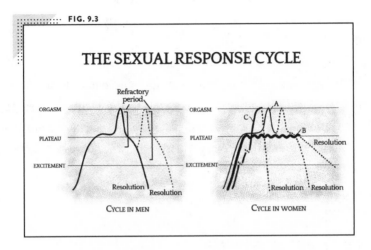

FIG. 9.3

THE SEXUAL RESPONSE CYCLE

WHEREAS MEN USUALLY HAVE ONE ORGASM, WOMEN HAVE
THE ABILITY TO EXPERIENCE MANY, AS SEEN IN LINE A.

Desire

Blood flow to the genitals increases. This increase in blood flow brings with it water, which causes an increase in transudate (the watery, viscous, protein-rich fluid) to the vagina. This is the "wet" that many women describe.

Arousal

As a result of the increased blood flow, the vagina becomes engorged. You may actually feel throbbing or an increased sensation (even if nothing is inside). At this point, the vagina becomes reddish to purple in color. They learned this because they used a rather interesting glass tubular dildo with a camera inside.

Orgasm

The vagina contracts its smooth muscle, which aids in conducting sperm to the top of the vagina where entry into the uterus can be facilitated. There was the same visualization with the dildo cam.

Resolution

With further sexual stimulation after a brief resolution, the vagina, unlike a penis, can maintain its relatively high rate of blood flow, which may be the reason that we can get back to orgasm so quickly. Having a vagina isn't all that bad, right?

More than thirty major brain centers are activated at orgasm, from the limbic system, which influences memory and emotion, to the hypothalamus, involved in unconscious control, to the technical area of the prefrontal cortex, which focuses on problem solving and judgment. This is why it's virtually impossible to say exactly what the "orgasm" part of the brain is. It's all of it.[26]

Orgasm Q and A

Question: What are the benefits to having an orgasm?
Answer: Not only is it breathtakingly pleasurable, there is supportive study that shows that it may decrease pain and quench fear and inhibition.

Question: How do I know if I'm having an orgasm?
Answer: According to the *Annual Review of Sex Research*, the female orgasm is described as "a variable, transient peak sensation of intense pleasure, creating an altered state of consciousness, usually with an initiation accompanied by involuntary, rhythmic contractions of the pelvic striated circumvaginal musculature, often with concomitant uterine and anal contractions, and myotonia that resolves the sexually induced vasocongestion and myotonia, generally with an induction of well-being and contentment." In other words, there is an overwhelming sense of pleasure leading to muscle spasms and then a complete relaxation of everything.[27]

Question: Which is better? Vaginal or clitoral orgasm?

Answer: They both come from the clitoris, just not the little dot at the end. Which sensation is better is an entirely subjective matter. The entire idea of the ever-elusive vaginal orgasm came directly from the Freudian view that somehow the vaginal orgasm is more "mature" than a clitoral orgasm and can only be acquired through hard work and study. Have an orgasm the way YOU have an orgasm, and don't worry about the rest.

FIG. 9.4

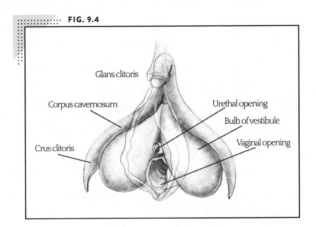

Glans clitoris

Corpus cavernosum

Crus clitoris

Urethal opening

Bulb of vestibule

Vaginal opening

Question: Does squirting make an orgasm better?

Answer: No. Female ejaculation should not be set up as some sexual goal or something to achieve. It's not like earning a badge from Girl Scouts; it's just a physiologic function.

Question: How do I squirt during sex?

Answer: See above. It probably comes from the fact that there is erectile tissue called the *corpus cavernosum* that contracts around the urethral Skene's glands and may express a bit of fluid. It is possible that the liquid emitted involuntarily comes from the Skene's glands on either side of the urethra, and it has no erotic benefit whatsoever.[28]

DO YOURSELF A FAVOR: MASTURBATE

In 1876, the French physician Roubard tacitly recommended the use of masturbation as a treatment for frigidity, or lack of female orgasm. He wrote more than a hundred pages on the physical causes of frigidity and physical versus "moral" (meaning psychological) treatment, and stimulation was actually recommended. Of course, direct clitoral stimulation was only recommended for women with a supposedly defective or undeveloped clitoris, so the physician had to diagnose a patient with some physical defect before prescribing such treatment. Before you think of these early French physicians as enlightened, also consider that the use of electricity similar to that of shock therapy was in that hundred pages of treatment, too.

You deserve to have an incredible orgasm, or two, three, or four, and until you know what works for you, no one else ever will. In addition, keep in mind that your orgasm and your sexual pleasure come from you. No one can give it to you. Our society has set up a system wherein men are supposed to somehow "give" women pleasure. We see it in movies, we see it in love scenes on TV, we see it in pornography. We see it everywhere. When's the last time we ever saw a woman enjoying herself on her own? Or at least if she's with a partner, doing something to herself to heighten her own pleasure? That's what I advocate. Wait not for what your partner can do for you, but what you can do for yourself.

Therefore, when you masturbate, consider what you've learned here. Your clitoris isn't just the small portion you can see, it is a remarkable neuro-erectile and neurovascular organ, and you must learn yourself how it works. Consider this: Try masturbating by stimulating those other areas of your clitoris, under the skin around and under that external "button," to see how it feels. Is it different? Then try masturbating with your partner. Maybe try stimulating the G-spot (the clitoral root) in addition to direct glans clitoral stimulation. How did that go? If things aren't erupting as you think they should, consider taking the Female Sexual Function Index (FSFI) quiz (see Appendix A, in the back pages of this book). In use for the past twenty years, this quiz has been used primarily in research studies, but just read through it and you'll get an idea of where you may be on the satisfaction scale.[29]

Remember, it *is* true that when everything is working well, sex is more pleasurable as a female because of our innate physiology. The clitoris is there for one reason and one reason only: to give us pleasure. Unfortunately, many women do not get to experience all the joy from the organs with which they were born, and I am of the belief the reasons why are primarily cultural and have been ingrained in us from antiquity. Should society be blamed for these outcomes? I leave that question to you.

DID YOU KNOW?

Primates, dolphins, elephants, penguins, bats, lizards, and turtles are all known to masturbate.[30]

10

Vaginas in Peril

Joan of Arc may have had vaginismus.

−DE L'IMPUISSANCE ET DE LA STÉRILITÉ,
DESCOURTILZ, 1831

What happens when your vagina doesn't work like you think it should? What happens when sex feels like daggers and putting anything in there, whether it be a finger, tampon, toy, or penis, is simply out of the question? It is extremely important to address sexual pain, an unfortunately overlooked and underdiagnosed condition that according to the World Health Organization affects up to 20 percent of women. Painful sex can affect all aspects of life, and historically has had some rather interesting diagnoses and cures.[1]

THE HISTORY OF VAGINISMUS OR VAGINAL CLENCHING

The most common cause for sexual pain is a condition now known as pelvic floor dysfunction, but throughout history, it has been known by many names. More recently, it was called *vaginismus*. But before that, the term was *frigidity*.

> **Fri·gid·i·ty**
> Pronunciation: \ fri-ˈji-də-tē \
> *Noun.* Being afraid of any interaction with the opposite sex;
> OR being sexually unresponsive, pokerfaced to his/her attempts
> to kiss/hug/have any interaction with you

Starting with canon (church) law in the mid-1500s, the inability to complete an act of coitus was a matter of law and grounds for divorce. Therefore, the need to correctly define it became paramount. Throughout the earlier centuries leading to Victorian times, physicians and practitioners of law, or sometimes both, debated on whether or not "frigidity" or "impotence" allowed one to leave a marriage. Remember, marriage was much of more a contract back then, and the production of heirs to inherit land or wealth was the primary goal. This counted equally for men and women. Unfortunately, whereas it was quite simple to define the inability to complete coitus for men (i.e., a flaccid penis), the definition for women was much more obscure.

Given that there was no physically obvious reason that pre-modern practitioners could find and thus no way to treat this condition in women, many resorted to calling it a moral problem, which had a complex and sometimes double meaning. As a result of the lack of a clear cause and effect, early doctors argued on several fronts. Either a woman's lover was bad, or the patient herself was physically defective, crazy, or had loose morals. This use of "moral" was a bit of a catch-all, and it could mean several things in the 1800s. For example, she could have been homosexual, or perhaps she engaged in prostitution, or maybe she simply failed to live up to her prescribed purpose as a reproducing female.

A French physician from the mid-1800s, Roubaud, toyed with the idea of using electricity, in the form of something akin to electro-shock therapy, as a possible treatment for frigidity. Keep in mind, electricity was new, and as with all new toys, people wanted to find more ways to use it. Dr. Roubaud found electricity "far superior to any other medication" (it's easier to just shock a woman pegged as insane or defective than try to get to the root of the problem in a humane way). Thankfully electro-shock therapy fell out of fashion, psychoanalysis evolved, and the debate raged on. The so-called "father of modern gynecology," Dr. J. Marion Sims, was involved in the description of vaginal and sexual pain as well, in the mid-19th century. Sims coined the term *vaginismus* and defined it as "an involuntary spasmodic closure of the mouth of the vagina, associated with such excessive super sensitivity as to form a complete barrier to sexual intercourse." He went on to state that vaginismus is a condition that is easily and safely cured with surgery.

Because an understanding of history is key to an understanding of our present and the formation of our futures, it's helpful to know that there was quite a robust argument surrounding what was known as "frigidity" back then. The word *morality* had very little to do with what we think of today; rather, "moral" meant some sort of mental problem or deficiency. And it's important for us to understand this association because of the bearing it has on us today as women.

French volumes from 1831 argue that female frigidity was more an issue of morality than a purely physical issue and argued against the use of surgery, favoring vaginal dilation and other coercive techniques. Other more barbaric and questionable techniques involved using ether or chloroform to render the female unconscious or using cocaine topically to completely numb the entire vaginal-clitoral complex. Although better than cutting the vagina open as Sims suggested, these techniques were probably either painful or ineffective or both, and some could be downright dangerous.

At the beginning of the 20th century, doctors started using electrotherapy to treat vaginismus. Even though it sounds like we're finally getting to something useful, like a vibrator, that is not the case. Physicians used long, thin, metal rods placed far into the vagina that were connected to a high frequency current. The electrodes were positioned at the back of the vagina. Since you are now a vaginal anatomy guru, we know that's not quite the right place to stimulate anything. Therefore, even though this treatment may have helped if placed properly, they were literally missing the spot. Not to mention the side effects! Patients could get shocked if there was a sudden break in the current, and with early electricity, that happened often.

The myth of vaginismus as a perfectly curable condition was perpetuated by Masters and Johnson in the mid-20th century when they indicated their cure rate was 100 percent. First of all, the cure rate for most things is rarely ever 100 percent, so you have to look at that with a critical eye. In addition, most modern gynecologists strongly disagree and find the condition to be a troubling, poorly understood, hard-to-treat condition that brings much distress to the woman and her (usually male) partner. Unfortunately, because this is a problem of female pleasure and one not completely tied to male pleasure and reproduction overall, research is severely lacking. Researchers have described vaginismus as a topic of "scientific neglect" because few research dollars have been given to this very important topic, even though there have been literally millions spent on tiny blue pills for male sexual pleasure issues. And even though we call it muscle spasm, we actually do not believe it's a real spasm, because the research we do have shows that reactive spasms of the vaginal muscle are not detected in the majority of women with vaginismus; rather it appears the muscles sit at an elevated resting tension, much like your back with improper posture.

WHAT IS VAGINISMUS/PELVIC FLOOR DYSFUNCTION?

FIG. 10.1

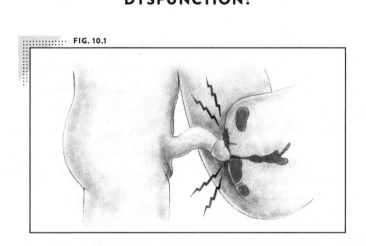

WITH VAGINISMUS, THE PELVIC FLOOR MUSCLES CAN CLENCH SO MUCH THAT NOTHING MAY ENTER.

Vaginismus is a condition that occurs when the muscles around the opening to the vagina are in something like a perpetual heightened tension, which often makes penetrative sex either very painful or impossible. The word comes from *trismus*, or lockjaw. Vagin-"ismus" is when vaginal muscles involuntarily tighten to a greater degree than the resting tension that keeps us from peeing on ourselves or experiencing flatulence at all times. Anytime something is about to be put in the vagina, such as a finger, penis, tampon, or a medical device like a speculum, the woman experiences tension and pain. It can also appear as itching or burning when sitting for long periods of time. Often women think they have a yeast infection. I see many patients who have been treated multiple times for yeast; they tell me they've done practically every internet treatment possible (see the chapter on yeast) and finally show up at my door. One touch of the muscles tells me it's not yeast, it's vaginismus. And this is the thing that often prevents women from having sex or causes pain during sex.

Vaginismus is in the category of "genito-pelvic pain/penetration disorders" in the *Diagnostic and Statistical Manual of Mental Disorders, 5th edition* (DSM-5), the definitive text on all psychiatric disorders that is updated periodically. Understandably, it's annoying that this condition is listed in a psychiatric manual, but it is described as both a psychological (emotional) and a pain disorder. Unfortunately, the true incidence of vaginismus is not known because women do not discuss their symptoms very often. We do know, however, that it's been around for quite a long time; it is not a modern construct, as we have learned from these early history lessons. It is also, in fact, quite common, with some studies of women evaluated in sexual health clinics reporting a prevalence of up to 42 percent.

Subcategories of vaginismus to describe patient variations

- Primary vaginismus: pain with attempted vaginal penetration that starts early in life and is lifelong.

- Secondary vaginismus: progression to painful vaginal penetration after some pain-free period.

- Situational vaginismus: inability to tolerate certain forms of penetration, such as penile intercourse, yet insertion of tampons or fingers is possible.

- Spasmodic vaginismus: spasm of the vagina.

- Complete vaginismus: inability to tolerate any vaginal penetration.

The definition of vaginismus as muscle spasms is doubtful because evidence from electromyography (EMG) studies doesn't show spasms on the tests. In addition, there has been a lack of agreement regarding exactly which muscle is the primary actor in vaginismus, but we're pretty sure it's the bulbospongiosus muscle, part of the levator ani muscle group. Vulvodynia and vaginismus seem to walk hand in hand as well. Several studies have shown that the pain of vaginismus is similar to the pain of provoked vulvodynia.

Many different organic factors can lead to pain of the vulva and vagina through a variety of pathways such as congenital abnormality, acute vaginitis or chronic inflammation, atrophy, damage to the vaginal lining from radiation, surgical scarring from female genital mutilation or lacerations during childbirth, central nervous system over sensitization, and even MS (multiple sclerosis), a condition of degenerating nerves. Often, these are undiagnosed vulvovaginal disorders. These organic factors combined with other factors such as anxiety, phobia, disgust, lack of sexual knowledge, cultural or religious beliefs, genital and sexual trauma, stress, and abuse, are all cited as possible causes. However, they are as yet clinically unproven, and the cause of this condition is likely some combination of physical and mental factors that require multiple modes and approaches to treatment, keeping in mind this may be a long-term battle.

The relationship between mental health and chronic sexual pain is complex and interrelated. Psychiatric disease is an established risk factor for female sexual dysfunction, including pain, and it is essential to distinguish individuals with primary psychiatric conditions from those who are developing secondary mood disorders such as anxiety or depression in reaction to their sexual pain. That's why your practitioner may want you to discuss things with a mental health professional. But it's not like this is 1850 and we automatically consider that our patients with pain are hysterics and somehow defective and want to apply electrodes to your vagina—we simply want to make sure your condition has been fully evaluated. Women suffering from vaginismus share a number of characteristics with individuals suffering from a "specific phobia." A specific phobia is defined as a "marked and persistent fear that is excessive or unreasonable, triggered by the presence or in anticipation of a specific object or situation." What if your condition is not purely physical? This is why it's important to speak to a mental health professional. Vaginismus and dyspareunia (pain during sex) are classified as sexual dysfunction that may be related to interpersonal and psychosexual issues, but putting the focus on those issues alone rarely resolves the problem. It is better to think of vaginismus as a pain disorder that affects sexuality than a psychosexual disorder that causes pain.

DIAGNOSING AND TREATING VAGINISMUS

We perform a physical examination to investigate strictly physical conditions, such as infection or inflammatory dermatitis, that may have triggered the pain. If a cause is identified, both the cause and the pain of pelvic floor dysfunction/vaginismus require treatment. As with vaginitis, the vaginismus will often resolve after treating the underlying cause. The most confirmatory examination requires both the patient and doctor. You have to tell me when it hurts. This is not a time to grin and bear it. If you feel pain under my finger, then we're probably thinking vaginismus.

Of course, vaginismus and vulvodynia aren't the only causes for pain with penetrative sex, so you and your doctor may want to work through other possibilities. This list is not exhaustive, but I just want to give you an idea of how many possibilities there could really be and remind you that none of them are your fault.

- Not enough foreplay
- Urinary tract infection or inflammation of the urethra
- Yeast infection (yup)
- Vaginal dryness
- Allergic reactions (spermicide, soaps, condom, etc.)
- Endometriosis
- Prolapse of the uterus (uterus slipping low into the vagina)
- Radiation therapy

- Interstitial cystitis (painful bladder syndrome)
- Cancerous tumors
- Bartholin's gland cyst or abscess
- Scar tissue from surgery or vaginal procedures

Current treatments for vaginismus are divided into four main categories: pelvic floor physiotherapy, pharmacological treatments, general psychotherapy, and sex/cognitive behavioral therapy. Of course, work with your provider to decide which is best, but I can provide you with some tips regarding treatment.

Pelvic floor physiotherapy

This is usually the first thing I recommend, especially if you're not yet familiar with how your vagina functions. These expert practitioners specialize in disorders of the pelvic floor and usually have the patience and expertise to get you long-term results.

Physical therapists use a variety of techniques, such as breathing and relaxation, local tissue desensitization, vaginal dilators, pelvic floor biofeedback, and even manual therapy techniques.

Primary and secondary vaginismus may be treated initially with myofascial release of muscle tension in muscles of the pelvic floor, thighs, and abdomen, with or without biofeedback.

Desensitization techniques are then applied to give the woman control over muscle tone and relaxation. These techniques are similar to exposure therapy; for example, when people who have a fear of flying do flight simulations and a deep breathing exercise or some other relaxation-inducing activity in preparation for an actual plane ride. The way it works for sexual problems is that during therapy, various escalating sexual activities that cause distress to the patient are imagined and are paired with a relaxation exercise. This way, as time progresses, the relaxation is what you feel as opposed to the anxiety provoking activity. Activities include Kegel exercises,

the pelvic floor drop technique (reverse Kegel), and the use of vaginal dilators. Self-insertion of dilators of gradually increasing size into the vagina
teaches the woman that control of her vaginal muscles can be voluntary
and, most importantly, painless. Desensitization is the goal of dilator therapy, not the physical enlargement of the vaginal opening. A small amount
of topical anesthetic should always be used on any object inserted into the
vagina because desensitization will not occur without painless insertion.

Pharmacological treatment

There are three main types of pharmacological treatment for vaginismus:
local anesthetics such as lidocaine, muscle relaxants like nitroglycerin
ointment and botulinum toxin, and anxiolytic medications like diazepam,
inserted into the vagina as a cream or pill.

General psychotherapy

A number of psychological treatments for vaginismus have been investigated, including marital, interactional, existential–experiential, relationship
enhancement, and hypnosis, all with varying degrees of success.

The first-ever randomized controlled therapy outcome study for vaginismus was conducted by utilizing a cognitive-behavioral sex therapy. The
treatment included a combination of educating patients about anatomy
and sexuality, vaginal dilation, cognitive therapy, relaxation, and sensate
focus exercises. Participants received the treatment for three months
either in group therapy or in bibliotherapy (book therapy) format. After
treatment, 18 percent (14 percent in group therapy, 9 percent in bibliotherapy) of participants in the treatment group reported successful
attempted penile–vaginal intercourse, while none of the women in the
control group reported having had successful intercourse. So what we got
is an approximately 20 percent improvement in the investigative group
and nothing in the other—not amazing results, to say the least.[2]

Other therapeutic approaches include shock wave therapy, sensate focus,
electromyogram (EMG), and biofeedback, but none have been evaluated in

well-designed studies, so we are once again left to throw spaghetti at the wall and see what sticks.

DYSORGASMIA

What happens when the very thing that is supposed to bring pleasure can also bring pain? This annoying condition is called *dysorgasmia*. This means, with the onset of orgasm, there is also pain, usually like menstrual cramps, but it can be quite severe. Although the condition is recognized in women, there appears to have been very little academic study—my search turned up only a study on men after cancer surgery—and therefore even fewer answers.

I had a patient who came to me with the strange symptom of cramping "even when I was just turned on." That meant she started to feel pain with only nipple or simple clitoral stimulation and had even worse cramping with orgasm. This sounds strange, of course, but there is a physiologic reason. Upon sexual arousal or orgasm, the pituitary gland releases a hormone called oxytocin. While oxytocin is a "feel-good" hormone associated with bonding and sexual pleasure, it's also involved in causing contractions during labor. Many women who have had a baby in the US have probably experienced a similar sensation when given the synthetic analog Pitocin to promote labor—and the cramps are fierce. In fact, many midwives and some OBs recommend nipple stimulation to help facilitate labor rather than this hormone.

Our unfortunate patient probably releases more oxytocin than most other women, which causes her pain with just simple sexual stimulation, resulting in quite a perilous and painful situation. Treatment? We're not sure. There have been some reports that giving women the same medication that stops lactation may help somewhat since the medication stops prolactin, and prolactin and oxytocin come from the same place. We're again back to the fact that research on women's sexual health issues is not well funded, so we're left with anecdotal evidence to try to help our patients.

MORE VAGINAS IN PERIL

We must not forget the heartbreaking practice of female genital mutilation (FGM) and removal of female sexual organs prevalent in some cultures. Although it has other names, such as female genital cutting or female circumcision, the result is the same. The power of a woman's ability to experience pleasure is diminished, and if that's not a vagina in peril, I don't know what is.

According to the World Health Organization, FGM (as I will write it, simply because I can't type the full term over and over without remembering my own personal experience of having seen it) has been practiced on more than 200 million women and girls worldwide. It can be found in twenty-eight African countries, in the Middle East, and also in Asia. Every year, nearly 3 million young girls are at risk for this heinous procedure.[3] Before you shrug your shoulders and skip to the next section, know that this also happens in the UK and, yes, also here in the United States. According to the CDC, more than five hundred thousand girls in the US were at risk in 2012, which unfortunately is the last available data we have.[4] The procedures often occur while "on vacation" with family members in their country of origin. Furthermore, while the UK made FGM illegal in 1985 (pretty late in my opinion), our country did not outlaw this practice until 1996. To make things worse, this 1996 law was ruled unconstitutional in 2018, leaving the states to enact their own laws. As of the end of 2019, only thirty-five states in our enlightened union have enacted laws against FGM.

And while you're thinking that it only happens in so-called unenlightened societies or third-world countries, know that a "cure" for hysteria in Victorian England was a clitoridectomy—FGM. Dr. Isaac Baker Brown, a well-known gynecologist of his time, advocated type I FGM (see descriptions below). His book, published in 1886, *On the Curability of Certain Forms of Insanity, Epilepsy, Cataplexy, and Hysteria in Females,* was controversial. But before you think he was alienated from his physician peers because of the grotesque, bloody, and radically unnecessary nature of this procedure, know that it was more likely due to the fact that male physicians were trying to legitimize gynecologic surgery as a true and separate specialty, and that insinuating that a psychological condition could be cured with a physical surgery was frowned upon. This practice was, in all likelihood, practiced in secret by his peers.[5]

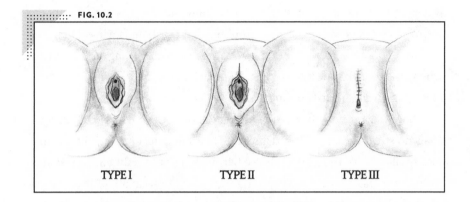

FIG. 10.2

TYPE I   TYPE II   TYPE III

HERE IS THE WORLD HEALTH ORGANIZATION CLASSIFICATION OF FGM.[6]

Type I, also known as clitoridectomy or *sunna*, involves removing part or all of the clitoris and/or the prepuce. This is the only type of FGM that actually could be called clitoridectomy.

Type II, also known as excision, involves removing part or all of the clitoris and labia minora, with or without excision of the labia majora.

Type III, the most invasive and severe form of this mutilation, is also called *infibulation* or *pharaonic*. It entails removing part or all of the external genitalia and narrowing the vaginal orifice by reapproximating the labia minora and/or labia majora.

This life-altering and occasionally life-threatening condition could result in many truly terrible effects, including infection of the bladder and uterus, scarring, fistula formation, perilous childbirth, and even difficulty walking. Of course, the desired effect is to maintain virginity until marriage—perhaps it liberates a man from ever having to please a woman sexually? Of course, these vaginas in peril could be helped. But I am quite certain you can conclude that there is neither the political will nor where-withal to combat it, this being a woman problem and all.

When I was a resident training in OB-GYN at a community hospital on Chicago's North Side, I encountered a patient who had undergone type III FGM. She was an immigrant from Somalia, and we will call her "Ayan." She was pregnant and in labor with her first child and she was perhaps about twenty-two years old. Ayan was genuinely happy about having a baby, it seemed, and smiled between contractions, only breathing more slowly when one hit. I was the first to see her, and when I went to examine, I knew something was seriously wrong.

There was nothing there. Everything was smooth. She had no labia, and I saw no structures that looked anything like a female, or even human. She looked like one of those genital-free Barbie dolls, with only a little V shape to indicate there would have been a vagina. Ayan's labia had been sewn completely shut some time ago, as it was a uniform brown, completely healed and flat. Her mother-in-law and husband were there, so I tried to keep a straight face, pretending everything looked fine.

The only way to do an exam was through a pinky-finger-sized hole where the vagina should have been. Ayan rubbed her completely round soccer-ball belly and breathed heavily when I tried to examine her. It was virtually impossible to tell how far into labor she was. When I went to report to my attending physician, he said we had to separate the labia our-selves. Since my attending doctor that night was male (the family did not want any male physicians), it was myself and another female resident who had to perform the procedure. We needed to separate the labia to show the vaginal opening and enable us to help her deliver. Neither one of us had seen anything like it, so we numbed the area as best we could with an injection of lidocaine and made a cut with a cauterizing knife in the area where we thought the labia majora should have been.

Once that was done, we saw something else. The place where a clito-ris should have been was utterly flat, unnaturally so—no folds, no hood, nothing. She also had no labia minora at all. At least we could tell when it would be time for Ayan to push, and she was a trooper, delivering a five-pound baby girl in less than thirty minutes.

After the birth, we saw she had a tear on the lower part of her vaginal opening. Her mother-in-law relayed a message from her husband (or more likely from her) that we needed to put her back the way we found her. I looked at my resident, another Black woman, and she looked back at me. There was no way in hell we were going to do that. We did a normal repair of the tear, and without even a discussion, we told the mother-in-law that since Ayan had just had a baby, she needed to heal from the original tear, and we could not put the labia back together without risking infection. It sounded plausible enough that the rotund in-law huffed but did not dissent further. We kept her in the hospital a few extra days to allow the labia minora to start to heal with the hope that it would be more difficult for someone else to reapproximate the original procedure, giving the scarring from healing. I remember feeling a profound sense of sadness when we saw the baby was a girl, normal and intact with labia and clitoris, knowing that one day she could also endure Ayan's fate.

DID YOU KNOW?

A major research website, PubMed, lists 393 clinical trials studying dyspareunia (pain during sex). There are 10 for vaginismus and 43 for vulvodynia. In addition, there were 401 published articles about vaginismus, 4,819 about dyspareunia, 843 about vulvodynia, and 3,680 about female genital mutilation. In contrast, the site lists 1,954 erectile dysfunction clinical trials, and a whopping 25,578 articles dedicated to the topic.[7]

11

Birthing Vaginas

I remember the shit, the vomit,
the blood, the stitches. I remember my battleground.
Your battleground and life pulsating. Surviving.
And I am the weaker sex?

—KEIRA KNIGHTLEY[1]

S ome of the questions that I hear most often from my newly pregnant patients are, "What's it like to give birth?" "How can your
vagina do that?" "How bad is my vagina gonna be after I have
my baby?" Having not experienced the miracle of birth myself other than
being the result of a birth (and a C-section at that), I cannot tell you what
the experience itself is like. However, I can relate my experience as an
obstetrician-gynecologist, and we can look to science to understand how
your vagina adapts to pregnancy, how she behaves at birth, and what happens or can happen to her after birth. Being informed is key to alleviating
stress and fear when it comes to one of the most incredible feats women's
bodies can accomplish.

WHAT'S HAPPENING DOWN THERE?

So that we may better understand how the vagina functions during pregnancy, let's return to her anatomy for a moment, and delve further into her physiology. Vaginas, like any body part, are not identical from woman to woman. Strictly speaking, however, the vagina is a tube, open at one end and closed at the other end. But it is not truly open in its natural state; it is like a pillowcase without a pillow inside. Remember the smiley vagina drawing from chapter 1? The walls of the vagina only separate or open when something like a penis, dildo, or other firm material is placed inside of it (air and the infamous queef notwithstanding). The closed end of the vagina surrounds the cervix, which is the opening to the uterus that allows for menstrual blood and tiny humans to exit the uterus. The only time the cervix opens up more than a few millimeters is during the labor and birthing process, when it dilates, softens, and shortens. In the middle of the cervix is an opening called the *cervical os*. The os is technically what dilates to allow the baby to descend into the vagina or for period blood/ tissue to leave.

Moving on to the deeper levels, the vagina is made up of muscle and other supportive tissues, which constitute the pelvic floor. It's also made up of glands and the lining, which is called the *vaginal mucosa*. Any organ that interacts with other materials such as food, stool, urine, and blood has a mucosal lining, and these have special properties. Mucosal linings must be able to stretch. In order to be stretchable, there must be flexible fibers connected in such a way that the lining can conform around another structure or material. Collagen and elastin are two types of fibers that allow the mucosa to stretch and then return to its unstretched state.

Researchers have made some interesting discoveries about sheep vaginas that we can extrapolate to humans. At the beginning of pregnancy, collagen and elastin are densely packed together in the smooth muscle of the tissue. As the pregnancy progresses, hormones are released that influence the way those molecules work together. Elastin, the molecule responsible for stretching, is made in huge amounts, far more than collagen. While this weakens the tissue, it serves an important purpose: to allow for stretch. After delivery, elastin decreases and collagen again increases, bringing back strength and reducing stretch. How quickly any given vagina is able to bounce back after birth depends on many factors, both genetic and environmental.

The same is true of the collagen and elastin in our vaginas. A healthy vagina looks more like the inside of the intestines. If you've had a colonoscopy, remember from the photos the many folds looking down the tube? Vaginal folds, called *rugae*, are useful for many things, such as holding moisture, maintaining pH, and allowing for greater frictional pleasure for all parties involved. However, with aging, lowered estrogen levels, and trauma from childbirth, the vaginal mucosa loses some of its collagen and elastin, becomes thinner, and flattens out (from its former rugae or folds of youth). It shrinks in size and capacity. The vagina also loses some of its blood supply so it looks pale as opposed to colonoscopy pink. All of these effects can cause dryness, irritation, pain with sex, lack of libido or orgasm, or all of the above.

FIG. 11.1

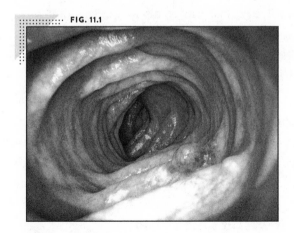

FOLDS YOU SEE ON A COLONOSCOPY ARE SIMILAR TO THOSE OF A HEALTHY VAGINA.

If you become pregnant, there are many changes that can possibly occur to your body, and, in particular, your vagina. Please remember that the following changes are normal parts of the process, so if you experience them, don't be alarmed. It is just part of the process of becoming a mother.

The Chadwick sign

The beginning of your pregnancy is similar to a low-level sexual arousal state. Higher levels of progesterone and estrogen cause increased blood distribution to flow to the uterus, about a pint a minute, to feed the developing fetus. As a result, the vagina and cervix will engorge and sometimes take on a bluish tint. You can see this quite clearly with a speculum exam. Originally discovered in 1836 by French physician Étienne Joseph Jacquemin, it was discussed at a conference at the American Gynecological Society in 1886 by Dr. James Read Chadwick. The American society promptly named it after the American, despite Dr. Chadwick's credit to the French doctor in his paper. This is why we call it the Chadwick sign— thanks to Dr. Chadwick (and Dr. Jacquemin) for noticing this.[2]

Transudate

Your vagina will also make more discharge. This discharge is normal— most discharge is, as we have learned. This extra discharge is a result of the increased blood flow to that entire region, resulting in what's called transudate, which serves to protect the cervix from infection and keep it closed. Transudate occurs when the veins literally leak out a little of the water in the blood. This discharge, or leukorrhea, may also taste more metallic, like blood does. Later in pregnancy, you may experience a sticky, stretchy, goo-like discharge. This is called your *mucus plug* and is an indication of the onset of labor; eek!

More orgasms . . . it's not all bad

You may notice that you have the ability to have multiple orgasms much faster and more easily, and you may find yourself better lubricated than ever before. Again, this is all due to that increased blood flow that feeds your nerves and that also, therefore, feeds your clitoris.

Tightening

In addition, you may feel a sensation as if your vagina has actually become tighter. While this is actually not the case physiologically, it again comes down to the fact that an increase in blood flow causes a change in sensation that is akin to throbbing, which many women characterize as "tight."

Lightning crotch

Your vagina may feel like it's in peril if you start to feel what the internet calls "lightning crotch." The medical term is called *round ligament pain*. The round ligament is found on both sides of the uterus and helps to hold it in place. As the uterus expands upward and outward, the ligaments stretch, sending sharp, stabbing pain that shoots to the vagina. While not dangerous per se, the pain can be so severe sometimes that it stops you in your tracks. Ways to combat it include avoiding heavy lifting and putting your feet up (let that partner of yours do the work), getting a pregnancy brace, swimming (zero gravity), and massage.

Enlarged labia

Your labia, both majora and minora, may enlarge due to the pregnancy-induced increase in blood flow. Your inner labia's increase in length may persist after pregnancy; they may hang lower and be somewhat floppier. They might also become darker (nipples too, they'll probably match), and this is due to the influence of progesterone. Unfortunately, varicose veins may also happen in that area. Thankfully, those usually regress after you give birth.

Bacteria

During pregnancy, the type and amounts of bacteria in your vagina fluctuate. In healthy pregnancies, the amount of the "bad" bacteria, *mycoplasma* and *ureaplasma*, decrease and *Lactobacilli* increase. There is some research indicating that if the vaginal microbiome does not change for the better in this way, the risk of adverse pregnancy outcomes may increase. Even in normal pregnancies, you may get bacteria in your urine and possibly a urinary tract infection. This happens because, during pregnancy, smooth muscle relaxes to allow for uterine growth. The same happens to the vagina and the smooth muscle around the urethra, where urine is expelled. Because the opening is more relaxed and therefore may sit a bit open, bacteria from your bum, like *e. coli*, are more likely to hustle up there and start to make a fuss. Your doctor will probably want to treat you to limit the risk of a kidney infection called *pyelonephritis*, which could threaten the health of your pregnancy. All the more reason to not let your partner graze your *e.coli*-loving anus upon entry into the vagina, no matter how big your belly gets.

It's itchy

Got an itchy vagina during your pregnancy? Well, we can usually blame that on hormonal changes and pH alterations that can change the vaginal flora, which of course is normal. However, if you are diagnosed with a yeast infection and you need treatment, know that the suppositories that are given are usually safe in pregnancy. There is some data that tells us that if your vaginal flora doesn't have as much *Lactobacilli* (remember the happy bacteria) you may deliver your baby early. Keep in mind, this information is somewhat new and needs more study to tell us what we can do about it, so more information is needed before you ask your OB for genital flora testing.[3]

IS SHE EVER GOING TO BE NORMAL AGAIN?

The best way to prevent vaginal problems later in life is to take care of it throughout your life and especially during and after childbirth. There are a few simple things you can do even before getting pregnant. First of all, hydrate. It's water that helps your vagina stretch. Also, try to avoid getting a sexually transmitted infection, which may affect your pH. We are also learning that multiple bouts of BV may be bad for pregnancy, so if this is a persistent problem for you, use a condom to decrease this risk until you want to get pregnant. You can't do much about the aging process or the birthing event itself (unless you choose a cesarean section over a vaginal birth), but these are simple things you can do to preserve the integrity of the vaginal mucosa so that it stays strong, healthy, and functional.

Of course, having a child vaginally puts your body through necessary trauma, and no matter how much you prepare your vagina for the task at hand, problems may occur. Some of the more serious include pelvic floor problems, urinary incontinence, pelvic organ prolapse, and fecal incontinence. Nearly 25 percent of all women and more than 30 percent of older women reported symptoms of at least one pelvic floor disorder, and most of these women had at least one child vaginally. Other studies concluded that between 25 percent and 75 percent of women have urinary incontinence, depending on how the condition is defined. Higher rates represent a symptom of occasional leakage, while lower rates are more likely to represent a disease. And unfortunately, simply being pregnant is a risk factor for pelvic floor problems.[4]

Similarly, published estimates of the prevalence of fecal incontinence in the community range widely, from 2.2 percent up to 24 percent.[5] As with urinary incontinence, differences in prevalence estimates are explained in part by differences in case definition, with some studies including involuntary loss of flatus as fecal incontinence in the definition and other studies limiting the definition to the actual loss of stool or mucus. This is how studies go, so we must work with it.

Trauma and injury in pregnancy and birth

Given the alterations in collagen and elastin, the stretchiness that occurs in the vagina also applies to the entire pelvic floor. This stretchiness allows all of the muscles and tissue to open wide enough to allow the baby's head and body to pass through, but this is still a traumatic event for your body. The more trauma there is, the more likely it is that the injury is long-term. The order of risk affecting long-term pelvic floor performance, from best to worst, is cesarean delivery, first-degree or no tear, second- and third-degree tears, episiotomy, instrument delivery, and finally the fourth-degree tear. Obstetrics has changed much over the 19th and 20th centuries. The episiotomy and forceps were once championed to save lives, both maternal and fetal. A Chicago doctor, Joseph DeLee, citing a persistently high maternal and newborn morbidity and mortality rate, advocated for a high-intervention birth, by cutting the vagina to decrease labor and using forceps if the cut did not result in delivery fast enough. It took around fifty years, but by the mid-1980s, research was showing that cutting vaginas helped absolutely no one, and it is now used only sparingly. We now know that a natural tear results in less trauma than a cut.[6]

The types of vaginal tears at birth and how we fix them

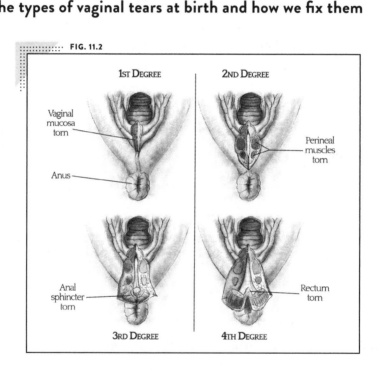

FIG. 11.2

TYPES OF VAGINAL TEARS AT BIRTH.

First-degree laceration

This involves injury to the skin of the perineum, the subcutaneous tissue, and vaginal epithelium only. The perineal muscles remain intact. We call this a "skid mark." We don't have to do anything to it, as it heals marvelously on its own.

Second-degree laceration

This type of tear extends further into the fibromuscular layer of the perineal body. Included are the deep and superficial transverse perineal muscles as you can see in the illustration. Most importantly, the anal sphincter muscles remain intact. This is the most common type of tear we see during a delivery.

Third-degree laceration

This is a more serious type of tear, which extends through the fascia and musculature of the perineal body and into the external anal sphincter and occasionally just to the internal anal sphincter. Incontinence could occur with this.

Fourth-degree laceration

This is the most serious type of perineal injury at childbirth. It involves injury to the perineum that traverses through the muscles of the external AND internal anal sphincter. This type of injury carries with it the highest risk of future incontinence of feces.

Each of these lacerations are repaired in a stepwise fashion. The extent and severity of the tear tell your doctor how many layers of muscle and tissue we must use to bolster the torn edges by holding them together with sutures as you heal.

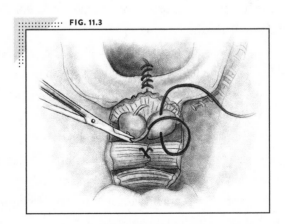

FIG. 11.3

EXAMPLE OF WHAT A PERINEAL REPAIR LOOKS LIKE.

PREGNANCY AND THOSE LITTLE LEAKS

During and after your pregnancy, you may get a little urine leak, especially as you get into your last month or so. Pregnancy and postpartum urinary incontinence are well-known and common aftereffects of childbirth. The hormonal and physical effects of pregnancy and childbirth are the major reasons for this. First of all, because you have more blood flow going through your kidneys, you have to pee more. Also, a giant baby head pushing on your vagina and bladder for many months doesn't help. Other symptoms during pregnancy include urinary urgency, urgency incontinence (that gotta-go feeling that results in an inadvertent leak), incomplete emptying, and a slow urine stream. These symptoms may also worsen postpartum, after you have your baby.

The increase in stress incontinence during and after pregnancy is believed to be the result of damage to the pelvic floor muscles and nerves supporting and controlling the bladder and urethra. As you know, the vagina is located underneath the bladder and urethra. Vaginal delivery is linked to a high rate of incontinence in the postpartum period, and women who may never have leaked during pregnancy could find themselves with stress incontinence after birth. The good news is that although during pregnancy many women may have a little leak, 70 percent of those will resolve within a year. We also know that women who had a natural tear had less incontinence than women who had to have a forceps or a vacuum delivery. So avoid the salad tongs and the suction cup if you can.

Many clinical studies have attempted to discover the exact obstetric event that causes incontinence. The usual suspects (please ignore the movie reference) include large babies and "difficult deliveries" marked by lengthy pushing phases with or without the use of vacuums or forceps. Unfortunately, no single clear event has been found to be the culprit, suggesting that postpartum urinary incontinence has many contributing factors.

Most studies evaluating the incidence and impact of postpartum urinary incontinence compare women with any urinary incontinence with women with no incontinence and do not include descriptions of the severity of incontinence, a major problem in the effort to draw appropriate conclusions. Remember, when we as scientists try to study a thing, we need to be able to compare like to like; otherwise, it's difficult to draw conclusions. This omission underlines the importance of using reliable methods of obtaining information regarding actual functional outcomes. The use of validated and reliable questionnaires to evaluate both symptom severity and quality of life is essential for future evaluation of postpartum pelvic floor changes. But, of course, we are trained to expect a little leak and just go buy panty liners or tiny diapers and contribute to the economy. That's why it's so important to study the causes and outcomes of these problems—so we can use the diapers on our newborns, not on ourselves.

NERVE INJURY

There is a complex network of nerves that feed the entire vaginal area, including the clitoris, labia, bladder, and even rectum, that can be affected during pregnancy.

One of the most important is the pudendal nerve, which comes from the lower back. It supplies most of the pelvic structures that maintain support and continence. As the baby descends down the birth canal, there is compression and stretching of the pudendal nerve that appears to be a major risk factor associated with subsequent diminished levator ani muscle function (the main muscle of the pelvic floor, the one you Kegel with). Other risk factors for nerve injury include the mother being a small size, a large baby, rotation of the baby's head during birth with forceps, and fetal malposition (breech position or if baby's head is facing up instead of down). Now, the nerve stretching may not be all bad news. There have been many case reports of women who report an intense feeling of pleasure during a natural vaginal birth. Perhaps this is nature's way of giving a little reward (other than your little bundle of joy). There have been some reports by women that during childbirth, they actually have orgasms. A French researcher surveyed 109 midwives who reported that of the more than two hundred thousand deliveries they assisted, around fifteen hundred patients either admitted to feeling intense physical pleasure or the midwives observed them experiencing what appeared to be physical plea-sure. While there's probably not going to be much more research on this (although there should be), we do know that orgasms can decrease pain, fear, and inhibition. Bam![7]

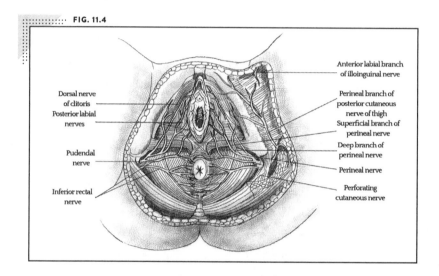

FIG. 11.4

Anterior labial branch of illoinguinal nerve

Dorsal nerve of clitoris

Posterior labial nerves

Pudendal nerve

Inferior rectal nerve

Perineal branch of posterior cutaneous nerve of thigh

Superficial branch of perineal nerve

Deep branch of perineal nerve

Perineal nerve

Perforating cutaneous nerve

THE PUDENDAL NERVE BRANCHES TO THE CLITORAL NERVE. INCREDIBLE
THAT CLITORAL SEXUAL FUNCTION IS VERY RARELY AFFECTED DUE TO CHILDBIRTH.

Occasionally, as a result of neuropathic damage and associated changes during childbirth, the pelvic muscles may fail to reflexively contract and help the urinary sphincter close during a cough or sneeze. The muscle tone diminishes as a result. This is when you may have to consciously Kegel when something is really funny. Some reports do show that the pudendal nerve starts to recover about two months postpartum. No excuse not to Kegel, though, and pelvic floor therapy may also help. While pelvic therapy after having a baby is standard of care in some countries such as France, we still struggle with this in the US. Postpartum care geared completely toward maternal vaginal care should be the right of every mommy vagina, but that's another book entirely.

ANAL/FECAL INCONTINENCE AFTER CHILDBIRTH

Leakage of gas or bowel after childbirth is rare but devastating. The reported frequency of incontinence of stool in women having their very first child ranges from 2 percent to 6 percent, and there are risk factors that you will want to avoid to keep it from happening to you. If you have a very severe tear, like a third- or fourth-degree laceration, the rate of anal incontinence is markedly increased. Anal incontinence is also associated with a forceps delivery.

Here's a bit of good news on childbirth and incontinence from the scientific realm: In 1997, Peschers and colleagues evaluated pelvic muscle strength by multiple modalities, such as physical examination and perineal ultrasound, before childbirth at 36 to 42 weeks, three to eight days postpartum, and six to ten weeks postpartum. They concluded that pelvic floor muscle strength is quite impaired shortly after vaginal birth, but for most women, it improves or returns within two months.

MY UTERUS IS COMING OUT OF MY VAGINA?

Years after you have your children, the muscles and tendons holding your uterus in place may begin to weaken with time and gravity. Pelvic organ prolapse (POP) is the protrusion or herniation of pelvic organs into or through the vaginal opening. The greatest incidences of prolapsed organs are directly after childbirth. The cervix itself can sometimes be seen peeking out of the vagina after prolonged pushing during labor. Pregnancy and vaginal delivery are the primary risk factors for POP. In fact, the weight of a baby as it drops lower into the pelvic region, laboring to bring the baby through the birth canal, and pushing the baby into the world all combine to weaken the pelvic floor and create conditions for a prolapsed uterus later in life.

What's more concerning for me as someone who has delivered babies is seeing the progressive growth in babies' birth weight over my years in practice. We know that harder labors and bigger babies contribute even more to pelvic floor weakening. Delivering a baby bigger than 8½ pounds can carry a risk of pelvic prolapse, so do your best to have a small baby (5–6 pounds is fantastic) by keeping weight gain to a minimum. Not all problems show up immediately. It may take years for problems like the bladder dropping into the vagina (called a *cystocele*) and associated urinary incontinence to show up. A *rectocele* (bulging of the rectal wall up into the vagina) can cause constipation, inability to completely empty your bowels, inability to hold gas or bowel movements, and even sexual dysfunction (the worst of them all). We also recommend doing targeted pelvic floor therapy to help decrease your risk and keep your vagina healthy and your uterus in place.

SEXUAL FUNCTION

Many women are concerned about how pregnancy-induced changes in their bodies will affect their sex lives after having a baby. While your vagina is made for stretching, birth trauma and the fear of the unknown heighten those fears. Know that minor tears and lacerations will have a very minor effect on how sex feels, but you may need some time to heal. Stitches, painful hemorrhoids, constipation, and continued bloody spotting are frequent occurrences that have the potential to negatively influence your desire to get back in the saddle. It all depends on your overall birth experience, so it's important to find a provider you gel with and who respects your vagina and her ability. The effect of a tear, referred to in the following study as "trauma," during a spontaneous vaginal birth can affect how you feel about sex afterwards. Trauma was categorized as either minor trauma (no trauma or first-degree perineal or other trauma that did not require sutures) or major trauma (second-, third-, or fourth-degree lacerations or any trauma that required suturing, including episiotomy).[8]

In a 2008 study in the *Journal of Midwifery and Women's Health*, women with major trauma reported less desire to be held, touched, and stroked by their partner than women with minor trauma, and women who required perineal suturing reported lower intimate relationship scores (IRS) than women who did not require suturing. Why could that be? I've spoken to so many of my patients who express fear and anxiety over intercourse with their male partners after giving birth and having a big repair. While they are afraid of pain, an even bigger fear is that it won't "feel the same for my husband." Maybe that's why the French pay for pelvic floor therapy after childbirth, *vraiment*? Do remember, MOST women's vaginas are able to regain most functionality after approximately two months. And you had a baby! That man should be so happy you chose him to mix your DNA with. You deserve some extra special petting after that. And even while your vagina is healing after delivery, your clitoris still works . . .

All in all, your vagina was built for this. During a healthy pregnancy, all the physiology, hormonal shifts, and pH changes work together to ensure both you and your new baby will be just fine. Having solid knowledge of what happens or can happen to you and your vagina can give you solace. Know your vagina will change somewhat through the process. Expect this. Roll with it. She's with you. Although pregnancy and childbirth are risk factors for urinary incontinence, uterine/vaginal prolapse, and sexual dysfunction in both young and mature women, it doesn't have to happen to you. In fact, postpartum pelvic floor and perineal changes are caused by many other factors such as genetic alterations of connective tissue, obesity, ethnicity, chronic constipation, even smoking. Prevention of long-term post-pregnancy vaginal issues is the cure.

Five ways to protect your vaginal health during/after pregnancy

1. Limit pregnancy weight gain to around 20–25 pounds. This may vary depending upon your starting weight and whether you are over- or under-weight. This will reduce the risk of urinary leaks during the pregnancy.

2. Have a small baby. Around 5–6 pounds is ideal. The concept of the "normal" 7–8 pound baby has seriously affected vaginas, especially in the developed world, where maternal weight gain can top 60 pounds. By maintaining a healthy weight throughout pregnancy, your vagina can be healthy after pregnancy.

3. Visit a pelvic floor physical therapist both during AND after your pregnancy. They can give you helpful hints to maintain your vaginal muscle strength.

4. Don't hold it! Try not to let your bladder get too full after pregnancy. Practice what's called "timed voiding." Go every two or three hours. If you can't manage that and need to go more often, try gradually increasing the interval between pee times.

5. If you can't meet with a physical therapist, try this at home: Flex your pelvic muscles (the ones used to stop urine midstream), contracting them and holding for about ten seconds. Do ten reps of this exercise every day. Work your way up to a twenty-second hold each time.

DID YOU KNOW?

The world's heaviest baby born vaginally was back in 1879. Anna Bates, a diminutive 7-ft 11-in tall woman, known best in sideshow acts as a "giant," gave birth to a 22-pound baby boy.[9]

12

Rejuvenated Vaginas?

They're all ugly. That's why we sit on them.

—ME

Labiaplasty and vaginal rejuvenation have been gaining popularity over the past several years. Prior to 1999, there were not many statistics on these surgeries. Since 2013, the number of documented labial and vaginal rejuvenation surgeries has more than doubled. Labiaplasty and vaginal rejuvenation are now among the fastest-growing aesthetic plastic surgeries and are probably here to stay. Since the ideals of beauty for female genitalia now include tiny labia minora (inner lips) and fluffy labia majora (outer lips), it's no wonder that so many women have asked me about this procedure—so many that I began to perform it. According to the American Society of Plastic Surgeons, as of 2019 there were more than 120,000 labial reduction surgeries performed for cosmetic reasons, and we haven't even touched upon the other part of the equation: vaginal rejuvenation. If you haven't heard about this yet, good—skip this chapter entirely and head straight for the chapter on toys for vaginas. If you have, then let's investigate and learn more about these procedures so if it's something you do decide to do, you are well informed and can ask the right questions (and more importantly, get good answers).[1]

WHY DO WOMEN FEEL THEY NEED THIS KIND OF SURGERY?

The term *vaginal rejuvenation* includes a hodgepodge of procedures and surgeries. It is unfortunate that this broad term has permeated the media and is now accepted verbiage. One procedure under this umbrella is the *labiaplasty*. The first documented modern use of this word (actually they called it a labiOplasty in the article) was by Hodginson and Hait in 1984.[2] The authors detail a case in which a 30-year-old woman complained of a lengthening of her labia, believing that this kept her from having an orgasm (considering what we know about anatomy, this was probably not the case). They described their new procedure as a "female circumcision" of the labia minora, thinking women might be more accepting of that term than the *-plasty* term, and the surgery they performed was very similar to one of the many types of this kind of surgery performed today. During my research, I began to wonder: If this procedure came about during the mid-1980s, then why is it that it didn't gain in popularity until the 2000s?

We don't have any solid answers and can only make educated guesses. Perhaps the seeds were planted back in the 1990s when Brazilian wax jobs, which reveal everything, became popular, causing women to examine themselves more closely once they were bald, vaginally speaking. Or perhaps it is the way women's vaginas appear in porn. Maybe it's the internet, showing idealized forms of female genitalia and causing women to aspire to that aesthetic. Some plastic surgery researchers hypothesized that a shift in focus in *Playboy* magazine from breasts to genitals influenced patients' emphasis on the look of the labia. It's quite possible. As with many trends, the media may have played a big role in the meteoric rise of labiaplasty.[3]

WHAT'S SHE SUPPOSED TO LOOK LIKE?

The female form has been scrutinized both artistically and culturally for millennia. In the New York Metropolitan Museum of Art, a full 85 percent of the nudes in their modern art gallery are females. Only 5 percent of the artists who painted works in that gallery are female, but that's another issue entirely. Although we know that the female nude is among the most depicted forms in art, the labia and vagina have not often been the focus, and when they are, controversy follows.

Why is something that half the population of Earth possesses such a taboo? My theory is that it is the fundamental difference between the male and female genitalia. Male genitalia hang loose and are easy to see. It performs by moving up and down, the testicles and penis can shake (if the male in question dances). Female genitalia is more mysterious, and it is this mystery that makes it taboo. The labia exist to literally guard the entrance to a most mysterious cavern—the vagina. Female genitalia and reproductive organs are hidden, tucked inside the body, and by virtue of that, have never been as well understood. However, there has been some amazing art to literally reveal the vagina to us all, demonstrating that the realm of normal literally goes far and long and wide.

Art has depicted labia and vaginas in both idealized and abstract forms throughout history, contributing to the controversy. From the very first known sculpture that depicted the vulvar shape, the *Hole Fehls* (German for "hollow rock"), to Georgia O'Keeffe's stylized design and everything in between, labia shape and appearance are a matter for discussion. The Hole Fehls, for example, was an amulet made from a woolly mammoth tusk and was likely used to enhance fertility. The figure's breasts and genitalia are exaggerated compared to its body, with large labia that appear to hang down.

Other artists such as Georgia O'Keeffe have chosen to stylize their depiction of labia (O'Keeffe actually denied that this is what her art represented). But if you know biology as I do, you know that a closed-up orchid looks very much like labia. And I might add that O'Keeffe did us no favors by insinuating that we look like flowers.

Pop culture took up this interest in the visualization of the vagina and its shape and size in the 1990s with the HBO TV series *Sex in the City*. In Season 1 episode 5, entitled "The Power of Female Sex," one of the main characters, Charlotte, has her vaginal portrait made by an influential artist known for these types of works. If you've ever seen the show, you know that Charlotte is the most conservative of the characters and having her vagina on a wall for all to see (which would have been expected more from the outlandish Samantha) was quite the statement.[4] Vaginal portraits have since made their way from the fictional world to the real one.

Consider this controversial art installation called *The Great Wall of Vagina*. Crafted by a male artist from the United Kingdom, it details more than four hundred plaster casts of vulvae. Measuring about thirty feet long, this polyptych is arranged into ten large panels and are unpainted, so you do not know the race or ethnicity of the vulva in question. The age range of the women is from 18 to 76, demonstrating that the artist wanted to include as many vagina variations as possible. The installation includes twins, transgendered men, mothers and daughters, and pre- and post-labiaplasty casts. If you check this exhibit out (it can be found online), you will discover the vast variation of vulva/labia/vaginas. Take these as a whole, and know that your vagina is normal too, because "normal" encompasses a lot. Like fingerprints, no two are exactly alike, even with twins.[5] There is no one true normal, and anatomy books should probably start to include variations, rather than a tiny idealized vagina/vulva complex. In fact, the website where this work of art appears states that "freedom from genital anxiety is the goal."

What is classified as a normal labia? Well, as scientists and researchers have tried to answer to this question, what they discovered was fairly similar to the *Great Wall of Vagina*. They found asymmetry rather than symmetry of labia minora to be the norm, not the exception. They found a wide variation in length, width, and depth, none of which correlated with sexual satisfaction. This means that those with tiny labia were no more likely to have a better sex life than those with larger labia.[6]

FIG. 12.1

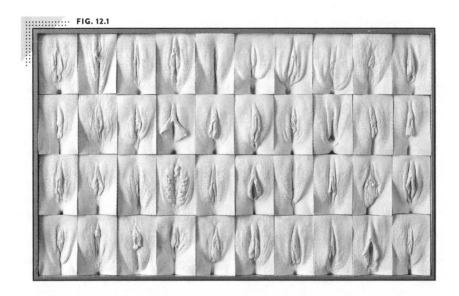

"THE GREAT WALL OF VAGINA" BY JAMIE MCCARNTEY

WHO SHOULD HAVE A LABIAPLASTY?

Ask yourself that same question and substitute, "Who should get their boobs done?" Or "Who should get butt implants?" I'm never going to recommend plastic surgery to anyone and am not inclined to get it myself, but I respect the decision of an autonomous adult woman who knows her body and what she wants. If your labia causes chafing or discomfort, or if your labia tears or tucks into your vagina during sex or become chronically irritated, then certainly there may be a medical indication for a reductive procedure.

The labia minora (inner lips), when measured from the uppermost skin fold to the lowest point, are usually approximately 0.8 to 4 inches in length and 0.3 to 2.2 inches in width. The reason that some are wrinkly is that the labia minora are the anatomical match to the scrotal sac, and this is also normal. Now, many of my patients tell me they noticed that their labia lengthened during and after childbirth and didn't return to their previous length. Childbirth is a contributing factor to a more lax and longer vagina and labia. However, other factors include simple aging, weight gain, menopause, chronic straining/lifting, or other chronic conditions such as Ehlers-Danlos syndrome, a disorder of collagen that can contribute to having labia dimensions on the upper end of normal. Labia length is not affected by sexual preferences or partners unless your play involves directly pulling the labia over extended lengths of time. The point here is that the labia can come in many shapes and sizes, and most of them are perfectly normal and beautiful just the way they are, but ultimately, the decision for cosmetic surgery is up to you.[7]

Many gynecologists decry labiaplasty as unnecessary, saying that plastic surgeons prey on women who already have enough anxiety about their bodies to get them to pay for expensive procedures. Certainly, there is the possibility of encountering a patient with what is called *body dysmorphic disorder*, a documented condition wherein patients are completely preoccupied with either nonexistent or only very small changes or differences in physical appearance. Their behavior is characterized by repetitive behaviors such as checking and double-checking themselves in the mirror. In addition, although they appear normal to the general population, such patients believe that they look abnormal, unattractive, ugly, or deformed. Those patients may show up at a plastic surgeon's or gynecologist's door, having already had multiple other surgeries.

Many gynecologists have chosen to not offer the labiaplasty procedure because the general thinking is that nothing is really wrong. Well, how do we determine that? As you now know, we have to look for the science and find the studies, and we have some recent ones. We know the overall prevalence of body dysmorphic disorder is up to 3 percent in the general population. Researchers have taken a look at who is seeking this procedure and examined their motivations. The numbers examined aren't that great, but it's what we have, so let's look. The first study to actually explore why women sought this procedure (not done until 2014!) compared fifty-five women seeking labiaplasty with seventy who were not. Measuring both psychiatric health and dimensions of the women's labia, they discovered that the women seeking labiaplasty did not differ with respect to anxiety or depression. They did, however, have lower sexual satisfaction scores, and ten of them met criteria for body dysmorphia. As a clinician, it is upon me to look at data like these while also taking each and every individual patient's request under consideration, examining her complete clinical picture and ensuring that her understanding is thorough and complete before anything is done.[8]

What about younger women and girls? Performing such procedures on anyone under 18 should be categorized not as female circumcision but genital mutilation. If you happen to be a teenager reading this, just wait a bit and live a little longer. If after you turn 18 your labia are still annoying to you, then find yourself a gynecologist and seek their opinion.

So the question remains: Should you have your vagina tightened, lightened, nipped, or snipped? The answer is, it depends. Many of the reasons I have heard for seeking this procedure have spanned from chronic pulling, tearing, and irritation to another kind of irritation: boyfriends' (usually exes) offhand comments. Most of my patients had been thinking about having the procedure done for at least a year, and about half of them told me their reasons were cosmetic alone. Reasons matter, and the decision is individualized and for adults only. I advise seeking the opinions of board-certified gynecologists who have chosen to perform this procedure. Ask them about their techniques and outcomes. Be comfortable with the fact that you will be forever changed. While you can have your breast implants removed, once the labia are gone, they cannot grow back. So don't have surgery, especially this kind, for anyone but yourself.

LABIAPLASTY TECHNIQUES

After the initial study in 1984, labiaplasty was the Wild West of procedures, with doctors worldwide practically learning by doing. The most updated study I found was from 2015, which examined nineteen different articles with a total of 2,204 patients, detailing eight different ways to accomplish labial reduction. Just to compare, there are only four techniques for breast augmentation. Most of the surgeons in the review article I found opted for what is called the *wedge resection* technique, done by making an incision that is "V" or cone-shaped. The natural edges of the labia are retained.

Some women and their surgeons choose the direct excision technique. Otherwise known to the internet as the *trim* technique, this involves partial removal of the outer edge of the labia minora and can be done in a straight- or curved-line incision by using either scalpel, laser, scissors, incising needle, or radio frequency (RF). This method removes excess tissue on either side of the labia minora and the edges are sutured together with buried, absorbable stitches that do not require removal. This technique results in an even appearance of the labia minora and removes the bulge between the labia majora.

Another popular technique is called *de-epithelialization*. This technique involves cutting an oval shape from the middle of the labia and then reapproximating either edge. The central de-epithelialization excision is more complicated than other methods and involves an elliptical incision to the inner wall of the labia through to the exterior side. Keep in mind, each of these techniques can come with complications, just like with any type of surgery. Because we want you to be as well-educated as you can be, know that bruising, scarring, infections, necrosis of the tissue, pain and discomfort, and hematoma formation (a blood bruise) are possible results of having this surgery. In addition, because this surgery has developed through a process of learning by doing, there is not much data to inform us as to which particular technique may give better results than another. But as the procedure continues to grow in popularity, the academics will surely follow. The American College of Obstetricians and Gynecologists (ACOG) has even relaxed its views somewhat. After completely advising against the performance of such procedures since their advent, a 2020 opinion statement acknowledges them. The statement encourages physicians to be aware of patients with body dysmorphia, provide appropriate patient counseling, and get the necessary level of training, acknowledging that more research is needed. I agree—our patients are demanding it.[9]

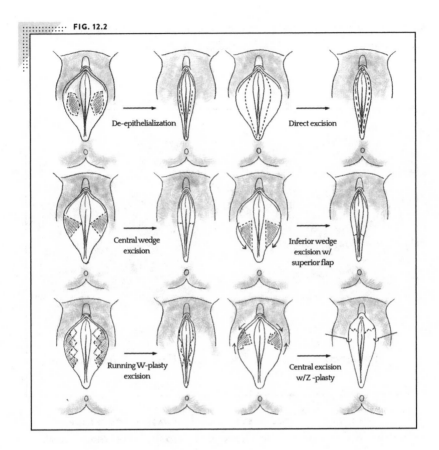

FIG. 12.2

De-epithelialization

Direct excision

Central wedge
excision

Inferior wedge
excision w/
superior flap

Running W-plasty
excision

Central excision
w/Z-plasty

VAGINAL REJUVENATION

I'll never forget a particular patient, let's call her Silvia, who came to me to have her vagina surgically tightened. After she gave birth to four healthy children, her husband started telling her that he didn't want to have sex with her because he didn't "feel anything" anymore. He even told her that he took a mistress! Tearfully, she asked me if there was anything she could do. I examined her, finding both a cystocele and rectocele; the vagina had begun to bulge out. The risks for this expansion and weakness of the vaginal muscles include not only vaginal birth, but also heavy lifting, straining when having bowel movements, and chronic obesity, especially around your midsection.

FIG. 12.3

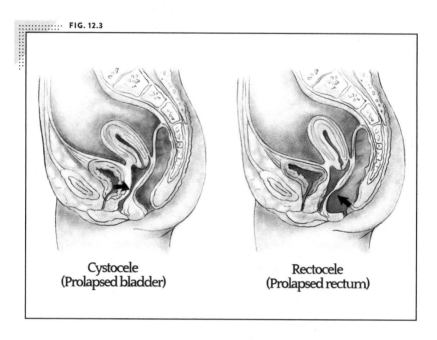

Cystocele
(Prolapsed bladder)

Rectocele
(Prolapsed rectum)

IN A CYSTOCELE, THE BLADDER FALLS INTO THE VAGINA FROM THE TOP.
WITH THE RECTOCELE, THE RECTUM PROLAPSES INTO THE VAGINA FROM BELOW.

A cystocele occurs when the bladder itself starts to bulge down into the vagina. Conversely, you get a rectocele when the rectum starts to bulge out from the opposite direction. Generally, you don't feel much of a difference yourself unless the bulge gets to the point where it tries to come all the way out of the vagina, or you yourself can feel it with a finger if you're standing or masturbating. Occasionally, you may feel a loss of sensation, especially if your male partner is on the smaller side. With Sylvia, my first instinct was to have her do an intense regimen of pelvic floor physical therapy, to attempt to bring the muscles closer together.

You may think that pelvic floor physical therapy is just those Kegel exercises you read about on the cover of Cosmo every four months, but that is far from the case. Imagine this: You pull a muscle in your shoulder playing tennis or moving a sofa, but you don't break a bone. You go to a sports physical therapist and they work with you to help strengthen the muscles. This is the same thing, just for your vagina, and there's no bigger vaginal tennis game than giving birth! These highly specialized practitioners are normal physical therapists who do extra training to assist women with the multiple issues that can afflict the pelvic floor, such as prolapse. Silvia agreed to try to work with a therapist. We usually recommend six to twelve weeks of therapy paired with home exercises, and the studies bear that out. We know that with an early-stage prolapse, performing consistent pelvic floor muscle exercises with coaching and supervision from a pelvic floor therapist can improve symptoms and lessen the need for other types of intervention.

In addition, we can also try what's called a *pessary*, a type of support that is worn in the vagina. It's placed where a tampon sits, and a woman cannot feel it once it's in place.

In the case of Silvia's prolapsing vagina, a pessary was a good option, and we offered it to her. However, her lifestyle and personal reasons made her shy away from using the pessary.

Many of the surgical techniques utilized for "vagina tightening" have been in use for decades, having been originally designed for vaginal prolapse, to repair a cystocele or a rectocele, and to repair a tear after birth. Performing this surgery on a normally functioning vagina without prolapse may result in sexual pain and pelvic floor dysfunction and should never be done. It is unlikely to make a difference in sexual function or aesthetics. However, if your physician has diagnosed you with prolapse, and if you find yourself unable to keep up the home exercises after you finish PT, surgery may actually be indicated and can be useful.

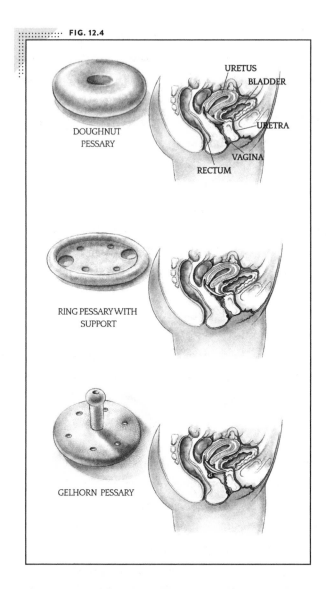

FIG. 12.4

URETUS
BLADDER
URETRA
VAGINA
RECTUM

DOUGHNUT
PESSARY

RING PESSARY WITH
SUPPORT

GELHORN PESSARY

**HOW THE PESSARY SUPPORTS A PROLAPSE. THESE ARE SOME OF
THE MORE COMMONLY USED PESSARIES: DOUGHNUT, RING, AND GELLHORN.**

How do gynecologic surgeons accomplish this "tightening"? Well, if you've ever had a vaginal birth and you either had a tear or your physician performed an episiotomy to help you give birth, you will have some idea as to what is done. Because most patients who need this type of surgery have some type of scar or laxity in that area, this is where we begin the work. We take a small, triangular portion of the excess skin from the perineum (the area between the vagina and anus) and then dissect and remove any excess tissue, moving in the vagina up toward the cervix. Then we put a finger in your bum (don't worry, you're asleep for the surgery), and reapproximate the tissue and muscles around the rectum and perineum. The bum finger is used to keep us from accidentally putting a suture through the rectum. It's a very important finger.

What if your bladder is the thing pooching down into your vagina? Well, we accomplish this repair in a similar fashion, just without the finger in your bum. With the bladder, we usually do not remove as much tissue, but the procedure is accomplished similarly. We make an incision in the middle of where the bulge is at its greatest and dissect off extra tissue. After removing the excess vaginal tissue, we then sew the underlying layers back together, therefore tucking the bladder back up into its proper position. Now, this repair usually doesn't last forever because gravity still exists and many women who suffer from prolapse have tissue that is not quite as strong. However, if the surgery is paired with targeted pelvic floor muscle exercises and you avoid putting too much pressure on your lower abdomen with weight gain or straining, it can be a viable option for many women.

After much counseling and conversation with Sylvia, we decided to proceed with a surgical repair. We performed the most extensive of vaginal rejuvenation procedures, a repair of both the anterior and posterior compartments of the vagina, while creating a new, smaller opening as well. The surgery went incredibly well, and we were both happy with the results. Unfortunately, her husband ultimately left her anyway. When I saw her last, she was picking up the pieces, yet still happy she decided to have the surgery.

If your self-esteem is directly tied to the size of your labia or vagina, consider the reasons why. Some of my patients who come to me for labiaplasty had been taunted by a (usually former) lover. Before you engage in what will be a permanent alteration of your body, consider doing this: Tell that unworthy human to bugger off and find someone who will love your entire vagina, hanging and free, and not some porn star–replica version of you.

DID YOU KNOW?

In a survey of more than two thousand women, 73 percent of Britons were worried that their genitalia were abnormal.

13

Toys for Vaginas!

We know that 70 to 80 percent of women masturbate,
and 90 percent of men masturbate, and the rest lie.

—DR. JOCELYN ELDERS, FORMER
SURGEON GENERAL OF THE UNITED STATES[1]

Masturbation, the act of self-pleasuring, has been around as long as humanity. You think that bottle of lotion in your boyfriend's bathroom is for his chapped feet? Now, you don't need a dildo or any other sex toy to bring yourself pleasure, just like your boyfriend and his lotion and right (or left) hand. However, I thought we might explore some of the wonderful things that are not your hand that we as women can use to literally power our pleasure.

Let's clarify a few things first:

- NO, you probably cannot get addicted to a vibrator or dildo.

- NO, you cannot "break" your clitoris by masturbating too much. (This is akin to the "going blind" myth that still permeates male junior high school locker rooms today.)

- YES, you should masturbate. Alone, with others, whenever the mood suits you.

- YES, you should try a toy. Not at your lover's behest, but for yourself.

HISTORY OF THE DILDO

That vast repository of knowledge, Wikipedia, points to a few ideas of where this rather odd word originates. They reference so-called "nonsense syllables" to fill out songs like "hey nonny no," or "hey diddle-diddle." That didn't seem like a good explanation to me. However, it appears that the root of this word may be lost to history. There is no Latin or Greek root, or any other root language that we would expect to tie dildo to any particular place. We do find a few uses of it in literature, such as in Shakespeare's *The Winter's Tale*. When referring to a rascally character in the play, Autolycus, a servant speaks this of him:

> *He has the prettiest love songs for maids,*
> *so without bawdry,*
> *which is strange with such delicate burdens*
> *of dildos and fadings,*
> *'Jump her and thump her'*[2]

This is Shakespeare's only documented use of the word *dildo*. The word "fadings" implies the "little death" of orgasm. The "jump and thump" should be pretty self-explanatory.

The Italians appear to have an early reference to this funny little word. One of the earliest definitions is found in John Florio's 1598 Italian-English dictionary. It lumps *dildo* in with other well-known euphemisms for penis: *pinco, prick, pillicock, pintle, dildoe*. So it appears that it really may have been a nonsense word, but nay, there is another possibility. In the 18th century, *dildo* was used to describe the small, round pegs that fix oars in place. In fact, there is a town called Dildo in Newfoundland, likely named after the boat pegs rather than the item.

Try another dildo on for size: The word *diletto*, or *deletto*, is Italian for delight, which some etymologists (those who study the origin of language) believe may be an apt derivation. Dildos can be quite delightful, no?

The earliest known use of the word *dildo* is credited to a bawdy poet called Thomas Nashe, from 1593. *The Choice of Valentines* is a quirky little tale about a young man who goes to meet his lover, whom he discovers has taken up residence (and work) in a brothel. He is so happy to see her, that just as she lifts her dress, he ejaculates, and it appears her joy is over. However, she proclaims (this is Olde English, so give it a minute):[3]

> *My little dilldo shall supply their kinde*
> *A knaue, that moues as light as leaues by winde;*
> *That bendeth not, nor fouldeth anie deale,*
> *But stands as stiff as he were made of steele;*
> *And playes at peacock twixt my legs right blythe,*
> *And doeth my tickling swage with manie a sighe.*
> *For, by saint Runnion!*
> *He'le refresh me well;*
> *And neuer make my tender bellie swell.*

Basically, she says that her dildo is more reliable, that it doesn't bend or fold ("bendeth not nor fouldeth") standing "as stiff as he were made of steele," gives her multiple orgasms ("manie a sighe"), and can't get her pregnant ("neuer make my tender bellie swell").

Whatever you choose to call them, dildos have been around for a long, long time. If you visit the Museum of Prehistory in Blaubeuren, Germany, you can gaze upon an eight-inch-long phallic object carved out of fine siltstone created as early as thirty thousand years ago. Nearly every culture throughout history has had some form of dildo.

The ancient Greeks worshipped the god Priapus, who is often depicted as having an oversized phallus. Their dildos were called *olisbos*, meaning "to slip or glide," and were made from leather. What did they use for lube? In an earlier chapter, we discussed NOT using things like olive oil as an intravaginal lubricant because oil destroys condoms, but in ancient times, you had to do what was necessary and olive oil was plentiful, so we can give the Greeks a pass.

The ancient Far East enjoyed phallic art as well. While it's not on display, the Metropolitan Art Museum in New York owns a jade dildo, about four inches long, dated to the Han Dynasty of China, between 206 BCE to 220 CE. While we can depict these treasures as art, it likely had but one use during its time. In more recent history, the Japanese depicted dildos in their erotic art and books. Beginning in the 17th century, these books, called *shunga*, or "spring pictures," showed women buying and using dildos as a tool for masturbation. Unfortunately, by the late 19th century, these playful sexual depictions, which also included female-female and male-male intercourse, were banned.

According to researcher Hallie Lieberman, the first modern-day dildo devices were actually made for men. Made with rubber by none other than Charles Goodyear (yes, the tire guy), Dr. Young's Ideal Rectal Dilator was patented in 1892. Dr. Young's claims that these early devices could treat everything from asthma (strange) to constipation (less strange) to addiction to masturbation (yeah, right) made very little sense, and were panned by the medical establishment of his time. While not sold as sex toys, these dilators were subsequently used to help treat women with vaginismus, which makes so much more sense to this gynecologist.

As opposed to your garden variety dildo, vibrators, by virtue of requiring electricity, were invented later. Much has been made about the story that 19th-century doctors treated women with supposed hysteria by using a hand to bring them to orgasm, resulting in the necessary invention of an electric or mechanical tool as their wrists wore out. Does this sound like a real possibility? True or false?

While you may want it to be true, and it may sound true, the answer is actually false. This probably never happened. Victorian-era physicians were unlikely to integrate orgasm into their treatment plans given the quite conservative moral beliefs during that time. If you surf the internet, you will still come up with this narrative depicting swooning 19th-century women being treated for hysteria with orgasms. This theory came from one place: Rachel Maines's 1998 book, *The Technology of Orgasm*. During her research, she formed this hypothesis and put it to paper, and the public went wild. While Maines has since publicly stated her theory was just that, a theory, you can still find it online as accepted fact. Again, to reiterate: Victorian women were NOT treated with orgasms. We, on the other hand, can treat ourselves, with our hand or with toys like our modern-day vibrators.

Although vibrators came to be in use in many countries such as Germany, Japan, France, China, and England from the late 1800s, they weren't exactly electric. Some were hand-cranked. Others used steam. The first electric vibrator was invented by a Brit. Like Dr. Young, Dr. J. Mortimer Granville claimed his invention was an essential cure-all. While he recognized that the device might be used for masturbation, he prescribed it primarily for men to stimulate their perineum and relieve them of impotence.[5]

So where do women come in? While men were allowed to be sexual creatures, women were not, and those who did express themselves sexually were widely disparaged. Sounds familiar, right? While "boys will be boys," women aren't allowed. These social standards unfortunately persist today. So even though women likely did use these tools for masturbation, the ads depicting their use had to be veiled. Not wanting to ignore a paying customer, the vibrator ads targeting women featured them using the product for "beauty" or when you're "out of sorts." In fact, vibrators have been receiving a Good Housekeeping "Seal of Approval" since 1953.

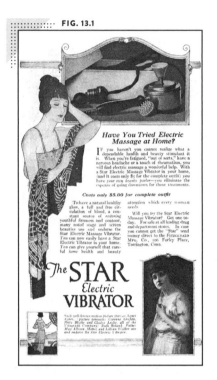

FIG. 13.1

A VINTAGE ADVERTISEMENT TOUTING THE USE OF A VIBRATOR
AS A "HEALTH AND BEAUTY STIMULANT."

DEVELOPMENT OF THE SEX TOY INDUSTRY

The sex toy industry is much like any other. It started with pure, American, idealistic capitalism more than a hundred years ago and has continued to evolve since then. In the days when Sears, Roebuck and Co.'s famous mail-order catalog was popular, sex toys (primarily dildos) were mainly sold through the mail. It was illegal, however, to sell such items through the mail due to an 1872 anti-obscenity law, so everything was kept hush-hush. Vibrators, conversely, could be sold in the open because they could be masked as "health-care devices." A penis-shaped dildo is tougher to pass as a health-care device and was deemed illegal and immoral at the time. In fact, the first dildos were strap-on phallic devices marketed as "marriage aides," to promote heterosexuality and male-female sex as opposed to homosexual sex or even self-love. Perhaps they feared that if a woman provided herself with happy, healthy orgasms with a penis-shaped device as opposed to a vibrator, then what role would there be for men? As a result, it would be many years before the opening of brick-and-mortar stores dedicated to the sale and promotion of sex toys for women.

In the United States, the burgeoning sex toy manufacturing and marketing industry was dominated by four men (of course): Ted Marche, Farley Malorrus, Reuben Sturman, and Ron Braverman. Beginning in the mid-1960s, Marche was an engineer and ventriloquist who, while seeking to help men, developed the first high-quality plastic dildo. Marketed directly to women under the guise of improving marriages and to doctors' offices for men with sexual dysfunction, it became an instant hit with women. Malorrus came shortly thereafter with a more cheaply made version and gained market share. As often happens in tales of American ingenuity, along came Sturman and Braverman, who bought out Marche's company and renamed it Doc Johnson. They figured the name "Doc" would lend legitimacy to what they were selling, along with their mascot, which was, of course, a friendly older doctor. Sturman and Braverman also put up brick-and-mortar stores. Unfortunately, these stores were not female-friendly, relegating women to catalog ordering, or slinking in and out of Sturman's male-dominated, peep-show-populated stores. This set the stage for a new type of store, geared toward women.[6]

THE FIRST FEMALE-OWNED SEX SHOP

The first female-owned sex shop, was (predictably) not in the United States. The history of London gives us the fascinating character of Mrs. Phillips. In 1738, she sold condoms, known as "Implements for Safety of Gentlemen of Intrigue" and was also known to have sold dildos. She was rumored to have taken many lovers, perhaps the reason she got into selling condoms. Even in modern times, the US cannot claim progressive ideas when it comes to female entrepreneurship. It was an enterprising German woman, Beate Uhse-Rotermund, former German Air Force pilot and mom of four, who began selling contraceptives through the mail in 1948. She built her first store, called the Sex Institute for Marital Hygiene, in 1962, expanding to more than twenty-five stores by the mid-1970s.[7]

The purported first female-owned and driven sex shop in the United States was called Eve's Garden. Its founder, Dell Williams, was a high-level ad executive in New York City in the early 1970s. As an active member of the National Organization for Women (NOW), she met now-famous masturbation guru Betty Dodson during a yoga retreat and she attended one of Dodson's seminars. Now, these were not lecture-based seminars—they were participatory. Upon entering Dodson's apartment, you had to strip nude. You then joined a handful of other women in her living room, and Dodson led you in anatomy, physiology, deep breathing, and then masturbation. Ms. Dodson recommended using a vibrator instead of a hand, and she used one upon herself, to the audience's applause as she climaxed. This gave Dell Williams an idea. Currently, the only way to get a vibrator was to go to one of the male-owned sex stores and deal with the shame, or go to a store like Macy's where a 20-year-old clerk might get nosy. She began to sell vibrators not only for pleasure, but being a member of NOW, to promote masturbation as a feminist and political issue. She started Eve's Garden out of her apartment in 1974 primarily as a mail-order business with a small showroom. Advertising in local feminist publications, the orders mounted. In fact, Eve's Garden is still in existence in New York City. Pilgrimage, anyone?

The presence of Eve's Garden sparked many other shops to open, and the business of toys has never been the same. In fact, in 2015, AMNE (Adult Novelty Manufacturers Expo) cofounder Susan Colvin estimated the market segment at $15 billion and projected the adult market would pass $50 billion by 2020. She wasn't too far off. The most recent statistics we have (from 2020) position the market for "adult novelties" at a little more than $30 billion.[8]

TYPES OF DILDOS AND VIBRATORS
AND HOW THEY CAME TO BE

No chapter on vagina toys would be complete without a full understanding of the modern-day development of and use of the vibrator. While dildos have been in use for (literally) thousands of years, vibrators are a newer invention, given the need for a steady stream of electricity. We know that early vibrators were originally made for men and co-opted by women secretly. And the most popular modern-day vibrator is no different.

Hitachi, the Japanese company better known for other types of small appliances, applied for a trademark for the name "Magic Wand" in 1968. It had (and still has) two speeds: fast and faster. Although the company never fully acknowledged its use by women for sexual pleasure, the box clearly tells a different story. Even dating back to the 1960s, the box has only a woman pictured on it. No men at all. One of the iterations of the device was called "The Workout," and the packaging showed women exercising. By the 1970s, the idea that the Magic Wand was for sore muscles was thrown out the window, and the box featured a woman wearing a cardigan unbuttoned down to just cleavage, just in case one was wondering about the intended use of the device.

It was the handy Hitachi Magic Wand that Betty Dodson, our masturbation guru, used in her classes during the women's liberation movement of the 1970s. And it was the desire to provide easy access to this very device that made Dell Williams found the first female-owned sex shops in the United States.

Thanks to Searah Desaych, proprietress of the sex shop Early to Bed, for contributing information to the following section about the main types of devices made to enhance sexual experience.

Dildos

Dildos are intended for penetration, usually vaginal. They do not usually vibrate (although you can add a vibrator to some of them). They have been around for centuries (one was discovered in 2005 that was found to be 28,000 years old!) and come in a wide variety of shapes, sizes, and materials. While many dildos look like penises, there are a lot of non-representational options as well. For soft dildos, 100 percent silicone is the safest and longest-lasting material. Porous materials like jelly rubber and PVC can harbor bacteria and may contain ingredients that irritate the body, so use condoms with those toys or avoid them all together. Hard materials like glass and steel make for toys that can put excellent pressure on the G-spot and create interesting temperature sensations. Glass and steel are also very safe material choices.

Vibrators

Vibrators provide a unique sensation that no human body can produce. "Vibes" come in hundreds of sizes, shapes, colors, and styles and can range in price from less than ten dollars to hundreds of dollars. Many people use them for clitoral stimulation, either alone or when having sex with a partner. Some styles are more like dildos in shape and made for vaginal penetration. Rabbit- or dual-action-style vibrators stimulate both internally and externally at the same time. Wand-style vibes can provide an incredible amount of power and look just like a back massager, making them super discreet. There are also toys that "suck" using new technology, and these can produce orgasms in women in record time. Rings with vibrators on top of them are meant to be worn by male partners to provide hands-free clitoral stimulation during intercourse (and can also be used by folks of any gender with a dildo). Vibrators can be made of hard plastic, 100-percent silicone, steel, or other soft plastic materials. Some vibes plug into the wall, many operate on battery power, and there are lots that are rechargeable via any USB port.

Anal toys

Anal toys are designed to be safe to use in the anus. All safe anal toys have a flanged base to prevent them from getting lost inside, so it is never recommended that you use a vibrator or other toys designed for vaginal play in your butt. The toys range from the very small (not much bigger than a pinky finger) to quite large. Most users start out with a smaller toy, and if they like it, they work their way up to a larger toy. Some butt toys vibrate but most do not. When using any anal toy, it is very important to use *plenty* of lube.

Cockrings

Cockring or C-rings are tight rings that people with penises can wear at the base of their penis behind the testicles to enhance their erection, in many cases making it last longer. There are also vibrating C-rings that are worn just on the shaft to vibrate against the partner's clitoris during penis-vagina intercourse.

Ben Wa balls

Ben Wa balls, while not a sex toy specifically, have been employed for literally hundreds of years. First referenced around the year 500 CE in Southeast Asia, they were small silver balls meant to be worn in the vagina to increase men's pleasure (of course). However, they were discovered to aid in pelvic floor muscle strengthening. Now, as a clinician, I'll say there is not much data demonstrating that these balls are better than learning how to perform Kegel exercises yourself, but they can be cute, and some even make a little chime. I figure a novice at pelvic floor exercises may get some benefit from feeling a sensation while locating and strengthening those muscles. An extra caveat I'd like to mention, however: Some have claimed these balls, or the related yoni eggs, if made of a special stone like jade, can "cleanse" your vagina or provide other health benefits. But I'll tell you now that they do absolutely nothing to balance pH, decrease infection, or anything similar. They may, however, look really nice on display. In fact, my mom had several jade eggs figured prominently on the credenza in our living room. (Ummm, Mom. . .?) Now if you just want to be fancy with your toys, you get the Dr. Williams Seal of Approval.

WHAT DO I DO WITH IT?

First things first: Find a toy that you feel comfortable using. For a first foray into the sex toy market, I recommend starting with something inexpensive, to play with various sensations and determine what you like best. A silver bullet is a nice starter vibrator, and it runs a little over ten bucks as of this printing. The classic Magic Wand is workable too. For a starter dildo, check out the Vision of Love. Always clean your toys before and after play; I use just plain dishwashing detergent. Careful with electricity; read the instructions of any new toy regarding use in and around water.

Next, get something to warm your devices. No one likes a chilly dildo. You can play with temperature as you get more experimental, but at least start with room temperature first. An easy hack is to wrap your toy in an electric blanket or something similar for about thirty minutes. If your toy is usable in water, running it under warm water works rather quickly as well.

Then, plan a time when you can be completely alone for a good amount of time. Find a comfortable place—some like to have a bath first or even masturbate there, with a waterproof toy, of course. Visualization of pleasure is important here. You have to know that what you're about to do will bring you an amazing sensation and that you yourself are worthy of this pleasure. Start with some breast stimulation, and when you're ready, fire up your friend. Perhaps consider not starting directly with the glans clitoris, but around the crus, root, and body of the clitoris. This is all dependent upon which toy you are using, but the idea is if this is your first toy, then take your time. As you climax, ride the wave. Don't focus on having another one, just enjoy what you have. If after you've come down a bit your body tells you to keep going, then do. Either way, great!

Although certain TV shows and movies have mainstreamed the use of toys for women's sexual pleasure, these appear to be a double-edged sword. One of the first mainstream peeks into female masturbation with toys was, once again, *Sex in the City*. A pioneering show during its time, one particular episode (Season 4 episode 8, if you're interested) features the "sexpot" character, Samantha, refusing to leave her house or do anything else until she can once again "find" her orgasm. She has a drawer literally full of dildos and goes through each until she finds the one she thinks will work. It is a little silly, and fortunately, the portrayal of the use of dildos has become more mainstream and not so heavy-handed. Everyone masturbates. We just have a little technology to help us along. A more modern example is an episode of the HBO show *Insecure*. The main character, played by Issa Rae, feels like masturbating, as humans do, only to find that her vibrator has run out of batteries. I like this most because there is no trauma surrounding it, no fantasizing about an ex and the like. It's just a human female (and a Black woman no less, because we do it too) looking to have an orgasm through some tech. And I say, Yahoo![9]

Women deserve to enjoy themselves at their own discretion. And I say, let tech lead the way and buzz on. Now, go forth and use your vagina to her fullest potential! Pause right here and go rub one out (or vibrate or finger or dildo one out, your choice). You can come back to this book later.

DID YOU KNOW?

In 2017, a survey performed by sex toy maker Lovehoney showed that 65 percent of vibrators were purchased by single women.

As late as 2017, the sale of sex toys is illegal in Alabama. I guess "Roll Tide" only goes so far.

14

Menopausal Vaginas

Wait a minute to do that Pap smear, Doc. I'm flashing.

—A. M., AGE 51

First of all, menopause is not a disease that needs to be treated. It is a completely normal part of having a vagina. Menopause is a part of life that is sorely misunderstood and stigmatized, as if it is the ending of a woman's life. In our modern youth-centered culture, women are pushed to remain young forever, and when menopause happens, like it will to half of all humans, we bemoan it. Every day I counsel my patients who find themselves at the beginning of the menopausal transition. Many seem funereal, others downright despondent. My goal is to encourage and educate them; we have cycles in life and one is no better than the other. In fact, it may actually be a time to celebrate. Life has given you wisdom, knowledge, and soon, no more periods. I encourage you to seek to understand and embrace these changes, because they are coming for us all. And with a better understanding of this part of life, you will realize that your vagina in menopause can still take you far.

Menopause was not always seen as a problem. In some cultures, women have been revered for the wisdom that can come with living life into menopause. In ancient pagan Ireland, when male and female dancers performed the rites to worship the goddess in the "fairy ring" circle dance, it was menopausal women who presided over these ceremonies. These ancient people believed that menopausal women had magical powers since their menstrual blood remained in their bodies, coursing through their veins, and did not flow out each month. Because menopausal women do not lose any blood, they believed their bodies retained their "wise blood" permanently, granting them special knowledge. As paganism gave rise to Christianity, the fear of these "wise women" possibly surfaced as persecution of witches, serving to fashion and solidify a patriarchal faith turning away from a female goddess-centered paganism. Perhaps we need to look to the ancients when regarding aging women and their sacred bodies.[1]

Most people know that menopause means no more periods, and occasional hot flashes, sweats, and other annoyances. But what I want to touch on is how we define it and how it affects your life and your vagina specifically. The accepted definition of menopause is twelve consecutive months without a period due to loss of the ovarian production of estrogen. "Natural" or non-surgical menopause most often occurs between ages of 40 and 58.

There are some situations, diseases, or habits that can affect when menopause will occur, although it is mainly genetic. A woman tends to become menopausal at about the same time her mother did. Smoking, chemotherapy, previous ovarian surgery, and ethnicity can affect the timing of menopause, however. Latina and African American women experience it a little earlier, while Chinese and Japanese women experience it a little later than White women, whose average age is 51.5.

WHY DOES MENOPAUSE OCCUR?

As we age, the estrogen production from the ovary decreases. This increases the production of a hormone called FSH (follicle-stimulating hormone) from the pituitary gland, which, as we have already learned, is a gland deep in the brain near the hypothalamus that is partly responsible for coordinating hormonal function. FSH is produced to stimulate egg production and ovulation. Therefore, elevated FSH levels (discovered via a blood test) can determine whether a woman has useful (fertile) or subfertile ovarian function or enough estrogen to produce an egg. FSH is low during fertile times because less is required to make eggs come out, and it increases as a woman enters perimenopause and menopause. Eventually, the estrogen level is too low to even produce a lining that can shed each month. Voila, menopause!

WHAT ARE THE SIGNS AND SYMPTOMS OF MENOPAUSE?

What are some other signs of menopause besides no bleeding each month? One of the first signs is the well-known and dreaded hot flash, which is a rush of heat to the face, head, neck, and other body parts—just one of the side effects caused by a drop in estrogen that occurs during menopause. The face may flush, and your heart may race. Hot flashes can impair sleep when they happen at night, which seems to be a common phenomenon and is one of my patients' most common complaints.

The lack of estrogen can have effects on other body systems such as the bladder, vagina, bones, brain, and breasts. Estrogen is essential for collagen formation, and this loss results in a thinning of the vaginal tissue, known as vaginal atrophy. Atrophy means the vagina is drier, the walls are thinner, and it can burn during sex.

Researchers simulated menopause in rats by removing their ovaries to see the potential effects on the vagina. In these rats, the concentration of both collagen type I and type III decreased. As you recall from the "Birthing Vaginas" chapter, type I collagen has a high tensile strength and type III is the most common type. Both work in concert to maintain a healthy vagina. As you enter menopause, these levels decrease and contribute to what we call the genitourinary syndrome of menopause (GSM) or the irritation that can result from these collagen deficits.[2]

In yet another study of "menopausal" rats who underwent induced vaginal trauma, the muscle strength, collagen fibers, and elastic fibers were all reduced or dysfunctional and led to an increased risk of urinary incontinence. So we know that in menopause these things are more common. Studies have also been performed on ewes that showed that vaginal dimensions increase during adolescence, peak during the reproductive period, and decreased sharply after the ewes' ovaries were removed to simulate menopause. Some may think a narrow vagina is a good thing, but a narrow vagina without enough estrogen to promote collagen and plasticity can result in a tight and painful situation.

Other possible effects
of low estrogen in menopause:

- Atrophic vaginitis
- Osteopenia or osteoporosis
- Achy joints
- Brain fogginess
- Gastrointestinal problems
- Thinning hair
- Facial hair growth
- Fatigue
- Headache

The rise and fall of women's sex hormones

ESTROGEN

What does this hormone do?	o Stimulates growth of breast tissue. o Maintains vaginal blood flow and lubrication. o Causes lining of the uterus to thicken during the menstrual cycle. o Keeps vaginal lining elastic. o Many other functions, including preserving bone.
How do menopause and age affect this hormone?	o During perimenopause, levels fluctuate and become unpredictable. Eventually, production falls to a very low level.
What symptoms may result at midlife?	o High levels can result in bloating, breast tenderness, heavy bleeding. o Low levels can result in hot flashes, night sweats, palpitations, headaches, insomnia, fatigue, bone loss, vaginal dryness.

PROGESTERONE

What does this hormone do?	o Prepares lining of the uterus for a fertilized egg and helps maintain early pregnancy.
How do menopause and age affect this hormone?	o Production stops during menstrual cycles when there is no ovulation and after final menstrual period.
What symptoms may result at midlife?	o Lack of progesterone can cause periods to become irregular, heavier, and longer during perimenopause.

continued

TESTOSTERONE

What does this hormone do?	Although known as the "male" hormone, testosterone is also important to women's sexual health: ○ Plays a key role in women's estrogen production. ○ Contributes to libido. ○ May help maintain bone and muscle mass.
How do menopause and age affect this hormone?	○ Levels peak in a woman's 20s and decline slowly thereafter. By menopause, level is at half of its peak. ○ Ovaries continue to make testosterone even after estrogen production stops. ○ Testosterone production from adrenal glands also declines with aging but continues after menopause.
What symptoms may result at midlife?	○ Effects of testosterone decline are uncertain.

SHIFREN JL, HANFLING S. SEXUALITY IN MIDLIFE AND BEYOND: SPECIAL HEALTH REPORT. HARVARD HEALTH PUBLICATIONS, BOSTON, MA. COPYRIGHT © 2010 HARVARD UNIVERSITY.

HOW CAN I TREAT MY MENOPAUSAL SYMPTOMS?

Menopause is an entirely normal process, and many women are completely asymptomatic or have minimal symptoms from the normal decrease in estrogen. A lot of women are not encumbered by the hormonal fluctuations that occur at this time, when their estrogen levels may rise and fall with the moon and the tides. However, some women do have reactions to this fluctuation and eventual permanent decrease in estrogen and benefit from some sort of supportive treatment.

Hormonal supplements can be prescribed to prevent or treat these complaints, but not all women need them or benefit from them. There are hundreds of studies that analyzed the issue of hormone supplementation, and the consensus is that each case must be individualized. The benefit does appear to be higher if it is started earlier in the menopausal process rather than many years later. And there are, of course, women affected more acutely by menopause and more treatment is needed.

Dry, irritated, and thin vaginas cause much distress and can mess up your sex life just when the fear of becoming pregnant disappears. How ironic is that? Vulvovaginal atrophy (VVA) or the genitourinary syndrome of menopause are the official medical terms for the condition. VVA symptoms include dryness, burning, pain, less lubrication, and pain with sex, called dyspareunia. Atrophic vaginitis is a result of inflammation in the vaginal area. While not infectious (antibiotics are not required), it can cause redness and (of course) discharge.

The following is an illustration of a normal vagina as it goes into and through menopause (when estrogen is low). The cellular architecture changes from a premenopausal state composed of primarily superficial mucosal cells, the ones that produce lubricant and are responsible for sensation, to being composed of those deeper layer cells called parabasal cells, with the superficial cells thinning out.

FIG. 14.1

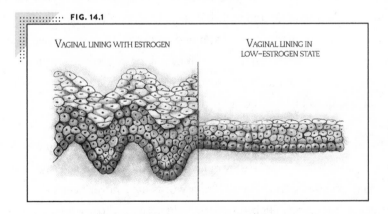

VAGINAL LINING WITH ESTROGEN

VAGINAL LINING IN LOW–ESTROGEN STATE

If your vagina in menopause isn't causing you any trouble, then leave her be. Remember, menopause really IS normal. Some women who are not regularly sexually active with men (or fingers or toys) may have dryness and irritation, however. If this is the case for you, then keep reading.

Things you can do
for a vagina in menopause

- Nothing
- Have as much sex as possible
- Regular lubrication
- Vaginal estrogens
- Vaginal preparations
- Oral preparations
- Laser resurfacing
- Radiofrequency treatment
- Nothing (really, it's OK)

Have as much sex as possible

If you are a woman who chooses penetrative intercourse, then please engage in vaginal sex on a regular basis. By having regular sex, your vaginal tissues are kept supple and well-lubricated, despite the loss in estrogen. If you abstain from sex for an extended length of time, your vagina may become narrow and the cells become thin, making penetration difficult. You may experience pain and even bleeding with sex when these dry, delicate tissues are possibly injured with the movement that comes with intercourse. You may even have some bleeding or spotting afterwards. What happens is a catch-22: Sex is painful so you don't do it, and when you don't do it, your vagina gets worse from lack of stimulation. As the saying goes, "If you don't use it, you lose it." Truer words have never been spoken.

I'll never forget a delightful 80-year-old patient whose primary care MD sent her in for a gynecologist's exam. She was complaining of some vaginal discharge, but had no itching, burning, or any of the other nuisances that we learned about in chapter 6. She just happened to mention to her doctor that she had vaginal discharge fairly regularly. The only thing significant in her medical history was the vaginal birth of three children. As a gynecologist, when you see an 80-year-old with discharge, you generally think of some type of infection resulting from atrophy, irritation due to atrophy, overuse of products, even vaginal cancer. What I saw on the exam was truly amazing. It was the healthiest, pinkest, most rugae-filled happy vagina I had ever seen in any woman over 50. When I told her that she was perfectly normal, quite better than average, I had to ask: "Do you have sex?" She said, "Of course, sweetheart. Me and my husband have been going at it like bunnies ever since he got that pill, and it's great. We do it at least twice a week."

Twice a week? This gynecologist's jaw dropped. Goes to show, a well-loved vagina will take you long and far.

Lubricate!

Lubricant is my first go-to recommendation for an irritated menopausal vagina. The lubricant rule of thumb applies for any vagina, menopausal or not: Use a water- or silicone-based lubricant for penetrative sex. An oil-based lube will suffice for masturbatory play.

Water-based lubricants often contain glycerin, which can dry out rather quickly in a menopausal vagina. If this becomes the case, add more water or saliva to reactivate. Easy to wash off, these are the lubes most likely found in your grocery or drug store.

A silicone-based lubricant is my personal favorite for a menopausal vagina because it does not dry out and is generally hypoallergenic. Don't use this with silicone-based sex toys, however, because silicone can damage them over time. Given its viscosity, it must be removed with soap and water. It's also slippery as hell, so if any gets on the floor, watch out! I use one of these for my hair (it's a bit kinky and needs the smoothness from the silicone), and one day I took a nasty spill from leaving just a bit on the bathroom floor.

I reserve oil-based lubricants only for masturbation or external play. Oil-based lubricants can destroy a condom's protection in under a minute and can actually contribute to dryness in menopausal women. I had a patient who had become sexually active with a new partner after being inactive for many years, and she complained that things were getting worse after starting out OK. When I asked her what she used for lube, she told me Vaseline. While Vaseline may be really useful for many things (I'm sure that could be a book by itself), sexual lubricant is not one of them, and it can easily contribute to dryness. Now, coconut or almond oil is OK for cunnilingus, as it is safe to eat, and tasty enough to add to the fun, but please avoid petroleum jelly for penetrative play.

Vaginal estrogens and oral estrogens

If run-of-the-mill lubricants still leave your vagina dry and unhappy, then consider using a vaginal estrogen-based insert or cream. Standard therapies include both topical and oral estrogen, although topical is much more effective for vaginal complaints. With longstanding vaginal atrophy, it may take four or more weeks of topical estrogen to see any relief, so stay the course if you and your practitioner decide to go this route.

The sooner a woman takes action to protect her vagina from decreasing estrogen, the better her results will be. The reason that estrogen is important for vaginal health is because it works to maintain the collagen, elastin, and robust blood supply that helps keep the vaginal folds or rugae healthy, juicy, and strong. As collagen and elastin break down and are no longer replenished, the walls get thinner and lose support. The vagina starts to shrink in length and caliber. The diminished blood supply only adds to the problem because a good blood supply is essential for carrying nutrients and oxygen and promoting healing and cellular regeneration.

Minimally absorbed local vaginal estrogen via creams or vaginal suppositories remain the endorsed treatment of choice for genitourinary syndrome of menopause (GSM) by both the North American Menopause Society (NAMS) and the American College of Obstetricians and Gynecologists (ACOG).

Will estrogen in my vagina give me cancer?

When I discuss vaginal estrogens with my patients, the first thing they ask is "Will it cause cancer?" The answer is, largely, no. According to a large multicenter study called the Women's Health Initiative (WHI), postmenopausal women who use vaginal estrogen have the same risk of invasive breast cancer, uterine cancer, colon cancer, blood clots, and stroke as those who didn't use vaginal estrogen. When used as directed, and if you have no other contraindications to using estrogen, vaginal estrogen will not give you breast cancer. So, if your vagina is bothered, use it. She will be so grateful.

Vaginal preparations

A new non-estrogen vaginal preparation has also been shown to improve painful sex caused by GSM or atrophic vaginitis. DHEA, or dehydroepi-androsterone (I know, it's a mouthful), is a precursor hormone that, when given vaginally, is converted to both estrogens and androgens (testosterone) locally. I find myself using this preparation for those patients who are still afraid of using vaginal estrogens. It does work but can take up to three months to do so, and it must be inserted every day, as opposed to the twice weekly dosing of vaginal estrogens.

We have some good supportive data for this treatment. Take this one published in the journal *Menopause* in 2009, when the makers were trying to get approval. They looked at 216 women ages 40 to 75 who complained of menopausal symptoms such as dryness, painful sex, or other irritation. After three months of inserting DHEA, they found the following:[3]

- 49 percent improvement in sexual desire
- 68 percent improvement in arousal
- 23 percent improvement in sexual desire

- 75 percent increase in the ability to have an orgasm
- 57 percent decrease in vaginal dryness

(These studies were standardized using the Female Sexual Function Index and Abbreviated Sexual Function score.)

Oral preparations

Oral preparations include a SERM, a selective estrogen receptor modulator. This particular treatment is a daily pill that acts to increase estrogen in the vagina while decreasing estrogen in the uterus. We know that using estrogen after menopause without balancing it with progesterone can increase the risk of cancer in the uterus, but with this delivery method, it's essentially a non-issue. Many of my patients like this treatment if they are uncomfortable putting something into their own vaginas. One nice side effect of this formula is that it may decrease bone loss. Different types of SERMs have also been used to treat breast cancer and osteoporosis as well. Additionally, a SERM won't increase breast density, which makes reading a mammogram less accurate. The only issue is that it can take a minute for it to work in the vagina, around three months. But stick with it, because it works!

Laser treatments

Most recently, CO_2 laser therapies have come to the forefront because of their successful use in improving facial tone and wrinkles, both of which are due to reduced collagen and elastin in older skin and women with low estrogen. So let's find out what role they may play in vaginas in menopause.

The word *laser* is an acronym for "light amplification by stimulated emission of radiation." Lasers generate light energy in the form of a beam of photons (light units). Different lasers have different wavelengths. The shorter the wavelength, the higher the energy. This helps to determine which lasers are going to be most helpful for what condition, which is why lasers for vaginas are different than those for hair removal.

Three physical characteristics that have made it possible to use lasers in the vulvovaginal areas are:

1. They are not ablative or destructive but have thermal effects.
2. They are absorbed by water effectively—the vagina is 90 percent water.
3. They are fractional, which means that the surrounding healthy tissue recovers and regenerates quickly and without discomfort.

In gynecology, there are three basic indications where lasers are starting to prove to be effective:

1. Vulvovaginal atrophy (VVA)/genitourinary syndrome of menopause (GSM)
2. Vaginal hyperlaxity syndrome
3. Stress urinary incontinence (SUI)

How do lasers work?

Laser treatment may improve SUI using the mechanisms of stimulant and photothermal effects. Laser light biostimulation of the cells helps to spur new cell formation. This may help improve vaginal functions such as secretion, absorption, elasticity, lubrication, and thickness of the vaginal epithelium, all of which are helpful not only for sex but for comfort. The photothermal effect is the result of the laser penetrating the vagina to a depth of 0.5 mm, resulting in a 30 percent increase in tissue volume. Thicker vagina, happier vagina. The mechanical traction on the surrounding tissues contributes to the production of new elastin and collagen. This, in turn, increases the thickness of the vaginal lining, elasticity, and firmness of the vaginal wall.

Atrophy of the pelvic floor muscles and the reduction of collagen content are important factors in the increased prevalence of both SUI and urge urinary incontinence (UUI) that can be common in menopause. Laser-induced neocollagenesis (new collagen growth) may improve the composition of the pelvic support tissues and help to improve overactive bladder (OAB) symptoms, that "gotta go" feeling.

There are controversies and doubts regarding the efficacy and safety of the CO_2 laser in urinary incontinence (UI). There are many supportive studies, but to date they are small and we need more.[4] What I've learned is that whenever something new is discovered or invented, there will be doubters. Louis Pasteur, noted Victorian-era French scientist, talked about these invisible life forms called fungi and he was soundly criticized and ridiculed at first. Same with Dr. Lister, of Listerine fame. Now we treat this knowledge as accepted facts. Insurance certainly covers your antifungals and antibiotics and will one day probably cover your vaginal laser therapy for menopausal symptoms.

How is vaginal laser therapy performed?

While laser therapy does involve the insertion of a small probe, the procedure overall is virtually painless, well-tolerated, and easily performed by clinicians. Usually, there are three procedures performed, separated by intervals of between four and six weeks. We laser each portion of the vagina in a systematic fashion, and the energy level chosen will depend on the device and the protocols established for each. However, treatment must be personalized, depending on the disorder to be treated and the patient's age and sensitivity to the laser. The only limitation after therapy is abstinence for about three days.

Lasers actually do improve vaginal atrophy symptoms

Improvement of vulvovaginal symptoms after fractional CO_2 laser treatment has been demonstrated in multiple case series dating back to the 1990s.

The results showed that either fractional CO_2 laser alone, estriol alone, or the combination of both treatments resulted in improved vaginal health and vulvovaginal atrophy symptoms. These results were reinforced with an analysis of the vaginal cell specimens. Meaning, it does work to improve a menopausal vagina's form and function.

We use the vaginal health index, or VHI, as a standardized way to determine the degree of atrophy in a given vagina so we can grade whether or not things are improving with our treatments.

	1	2	3	4	5
Elasticity	None	Poor	Fair	Good	Excellent
Fluid volume	None	Scant amount, vault not entirely covered	Superficial amount, vault entirely covered	Moderate amount	Normal amount
pH	6.1 or above	5.6–6.0	5.1–5.5	4.7–5.0	4.6 or below
Epithelial integrity	Petechiae noted before contact	Bleeds with light contact	Bleeds with scraping	Not friable thin epithelium	Normal
Moisture	None, surface inflamed	None, surface not inflamed	Minimal	Moderate	Normal

PACE, RAFFAELA & PORTUESI, ROSALBA. (2018). VAGINAL HEALTH INDEX SCORE AND UROGENITAL SYNDROME OF MENOPAUSE. GAZZETTA MEDICA ITALIANA ARCHIVIO PER LE SCIENZE MEDICHE. 177. 10.23736/S0393-3660.18.03686-0.

What researchers have found is that the combined use of laser and estrogen resulted in improvement of the vaginal health index after eight weeks. Sokol and Karram, some of the pioneers in the vaginal laser space, evaluated the efficiency and safety of fractional CO_2 laser for VVA one year after treatment and demonstrated that the positive effects on VVA symptoms (burning, dryness, and dyspareunia) and VHI persisted for an entire year after three sessions of fractional CO_2 laser. These long-term results show us that this technology is useful and can improve quality of life and overall satisfaction.

Lasers for sexual satisfaction studies

Lasers appear to have a positive effect on menopausal sexual satisfaction. Politano and colleagues evaluated seventy-two postmenopausal women who were randomly put into three different treatment groups: CO_2 laser, estrogen cream, and vaginal lubricant. Vaginal maturation, Vaginal Health Index (VHI) score, and Female Sexual Function Index (FSFI) were evaluated before treatment and after fourteen weeks of therapy. The results showed an improvement in the vaginal elasticity, volume, moisture, and pH in the CO_2 laser and estrogen cream groups. Cells also appeared more developed, which indicates an improvement in tissue thickness. Thicker vagina = happy vagina.

Other researchers looked at overall satisfaction even more specifically. Their data indicated a significant improvement in VVA symptoms (vaginal dryness, burning, itching, and dyspareunia) in patients who had undergone three sessions of vaginal fractional CO_2 laser treatment. Overall, 91.7 percent of patients were satisfied or very satisfied with the procedure and experienced considerable improvement in quality of life, which includes sexual satisfaction. Also, no adverse events like infection or burns due to fractional CO_2 laser treatment occurred. It's time to have the laser covered by insurance. Unfortunately, things that improve women's sex lives are usually not covered. I have a friend who works for a company that treats Peyronie's disease (crooked penises) and her treatment, which involves directly injecting the penis, is completely covered. And a pain-free laser with demonstrable effects is not? The irony is not lost on us, because we know who is making those decisions on what gets covered and what does not.

GET YOUR MENOPAUSAL VAGINA INTO SHAPE WITH SOME EXERCISE

Because we know that estrogen helps to maintain the muscle tone around the vagina, we can surmise that the loss of estrogen that starts at perimenopause and continues through the menopausal period contributes to a weakening of the muscles through the entire body, so we need to pay attention to the muscles. But since we're a vagina book here, let's focus on that. Menopause can worsen a pelvic floor already weakened from childbirth, weight gain, smoker's cough, or even chronic constipation, which can cause those little leaks of urine or even result in the uterus or vagina falling out. This is called pelvic muscle and vaginal laxity. We also know that according to Masters and Johnson, sexual satisfaction is directly correlated with the amount of frictional forces generated during coitus.[5] That friction can increase the pressure on the clitoris's G-spot and therefore increase feminine vaginal/clitoral pleasure. Conversely, less friction can result in less pressure and less pleasure in turn.

Signs of vaginal laxity include:

- Leakage of urine with coughing/sneezing/laughing
- Feeling of "heaviness" in the pelvis
- Chronic lower pelvic pain
- Pressure in the vagina
- Difficulty passing a bowel movement
  or having to put a finger in the vagina to press it out
- Increased urinary frequency or urinary tract infections

Should I exercise, you ask? Yes—you'll need more than Kegels, but Kegels do play a part. Key thing: You don't need to buy a single thing to perform any of these exercises. No Ben Wa balls, no tension straps, no teas to steam, no nothing. Just you, some focus, and your vagina. There are three exercises you can do at home that cost no money and will absolutely help.

Kegels: tried and true

The studies continue to confirm it: Routine and consistent Kegel muscle exercises improve sexual function and even decrease stress incontinence leaks.

How to do them: Visualize the area between your vagina and anus, the perineum. Imagine pulling those muscles upward toward your head, as if you were trying to stop your urine stream or even stop passing gas. You do not have to be lying down. In fact, I do a Kegel myself every time I prompt my patients to do one during our annual pelvic exams.

A little poem about doing Kegels:

> *You can do them in your bed.*
> *You can do them on your head.*
> *You can do them on your knees*
> *You can do them climbing trees*
> *You can do them and clean your room*
> *You can do them with pan and broom.*
> *You can do them, Sam-I-Am,*
> *You can do them, yes you can!*

FIG. 14.2

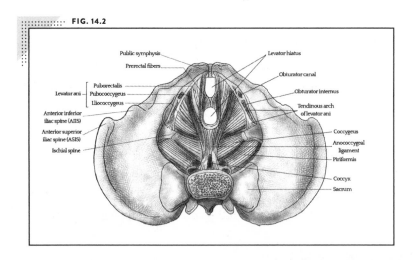

THESE ARE THE MUSCLES WITH WHICH YOU KEGEL—PUBORECTALIS, PUBOCOCCYGEUS, AND ILIOCOCCYGEUS—THE LEVATOR ANI MUSCLE GROUP.

I recommend at least ten sets of ten repetitions of vaginal muscle contractions lasting five to ten seconds each, every day for at least eight weeks. Then maintain at five sets of five reps a day, forever. This is where my patients have trouble, keeping up with doing the exercises every single day. Once you start, don't slow down as soon as you start feeling better. That's when it's time to keep it up and double down on the pull-ups. Again, this is totally free of charge and has very good efficacy. Studies show that postmenopausal women who regularly perform Kegel exercises registered more sexual arousal than those who do not.[6]

Small note: Don't do these while you're urinating; it could actually cause incomplete bladder emptying and lead to urinary tract infections in the long term.

Squats: not just for your bum

Aside from being one of the most natural ways to deliver a child, squats can be an excellent long-term way to help strengthen your pelvic floor. However, don't just start squatting down and expect amazing results. Most of us don't remember how to squat properly, and it can really do a number on your back if not performed correctly. Here are a few hints to perform it right:

- Start with your feet shoulder width apart.

- Keep your heels down.

- Keep your back straight and only lean slightly forward.

- Imagine keeping your head perfectly balanced and in the center of gravity.

- Once you're in the squat, don't bear down (you're not having a baby now).

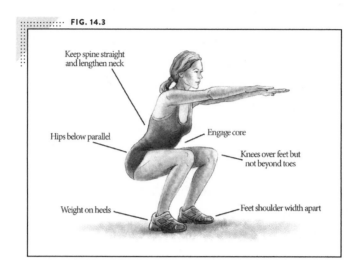

FIG. 14.3

Keep spine straight
and lengthen neck

Hips below parallel

Engage core

Knees over feet but
not beyond toes

Weight on heels

Feet shoulder width apart

THE PROPER FORM FOR A SQUAT EXERCISE. NOTE THE BACK REMAINS STRAIGHT, FEET ARE PARALLEL, AND THE CORE IS ENGAGED.

If you have very small children in your life, watch them squat. They really know how to do it, and they do it a lot. It's a natural position for them, as it once was for us. In fact, in many Southeast Asian cultures, adults still squat regularly, either as a chair substitute or for toileting. The first time I went to Japan and saw that the public toilet was flush (ha) with the ground, I had a time! But once you get the hang of doing squats, it can be fantastic for your overall pelvic (and therefore vaginal) health. And yes, they also strengthen your butt muscles, and because good butts are a thing, have at it. Do these ten times a day, forever.

Bridge pose

While this is a well-known yoga pose called the Setu Bandhasana, the bridge hold can help elevate and support your pelvic floor. Although we don't have as many studies for yoga poses as we do for traditional Kegel muscle exercises, the muscles that are engaged in this pose all work to support your core and pelvic muscles; having done this pose myself, I find it a helpful addition.

It is not for those with any back or neck problems, however, so make sure to talk to your practitioner before including this in your regimen. Start by lying flat on your back on the floor on a mat or carpet; not your bed, it's too mushy. Unlike Kegels, which you can do randomly and no one knows, and squats, which you could get away with doing in your office, the bridge might best be done at home, in concert with some slow and deep breaths to help with pelvic relaxation.

How to do the bridge:[7]

- Lie flat on your back and bring your knees up with your feet on the floor, parallel with one another and about the same width apart as your hips. Leave your arms flat at your sides.

- Keep your knees over your heels, and lift your buttocks up. Keep your feet flat on the floor. Start with a small lift, say around 2–3 inches at first, and work toward bringing your bottom up until your thighs are almost parallel to the floor.

- Push your knees forward and lengthen your tailbone (tuck your pelvis under). Start with holding this position for about four seconds, then lower your hips and rest. Work your way up to thirty seconds.

FIG. 14.4

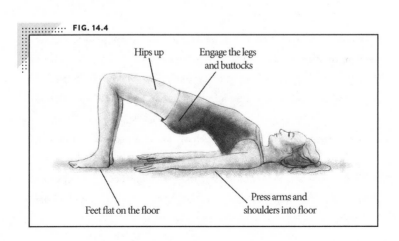

Hips up

Engage the legs and buttocks

Feet flat on the floor

Press arms and shoulders into floor

ILLUSTRATION OF BRIDGE POSE.

Menopausal vagina patient's FAQs

- **How long will I be in menopause?** Technically, you are menopausal from twelve months after your last period until forever. Some people call this postmenopause. How long you may have some of the bothersome symptoms of menopause varies, but this averages six months to two years. In rare instances, women may have hot flashes for ten years or more.

- **Are there any herbs known to help menopausal vaginal symptoms?** Currently, we do not have enough data to recommend any herbal vaginal preparation. Again, please discuss any inserts with your practitioner before trying.

- **I'm not sexually active right now. What should I do?** Absolutely nothing, if you aren't having any vaginal symptoms.

- **I haven't been sexually active for many years since menopause, but I'm interested now. Do you have any recommendations?** That depends. Give sex a try first, and if you find it to not be as comfortable and as pleasurable as you remember, then start with the basics: lubricant and great foreplay. If that's not doing it, then talk with a gynecologist who may make some other recommendations like those mentioned in the chapter.

- **Are bioidentical hormones better for my menopausal vagina than regular ones?** Bioidentical hormones began as a marketing term indicating medication that has been individualized for a specific patient and compounded by a specialty pharmacy. Now we describe these formulas as having a similar molecular structure as the hormones found in the body. If you have found a pre-made, off-the-shelf formula that works well for you, there is no need to believe that bioidenticals are somehow better; they have not been proven to be safer. Work with your practitioner to determine what may be best for you.

- **How long should I take hormones for menopause?** Traditional hormone therapy is indicated for hot flashes in menopause, and it should be taken primarily for that concern. Most women take hormone therapy for about two years, but I have some patients who have continued for up to ten. This should be monitored and individualized with your practitioner. Vaginal treatments, conversely, can be used as long as they are needed.

DID YOU KNOW?

The first estrogen treatment for menopause came out in 1942. It was extracted from pregnant mare urine, resulting in its name: Premarin®. At the height of its popularity, sales of this drug exceeded $1 billion.

15

Vaginalism: Vaginas in Race and Culture

You may write me down in history
With your bitter, twisted lies,
You may trod me in the very dirt
But still, like dust, I'll rise.

—MAYA ANGELOU

When I sat down to write this chapter, it was my goal to address some of the social aspects of vaginalism (yes, I just made up a word) that I have personally noticed over the years. However, as I continued to research, talking to women and learning more about this rather touchy subject, I decided to explore this topic once more from a historical context and gradually bring our discussion to the modern day. In this way, we can deepen our overall understanding of feminism more broadly from a cultural standpoint and vaginalism more specifically from a racial and socioeconomic point of view. It is my hope that as vagina knowledge is elevated, the -isms that affect our vaginas, such as sexism and racism, will start to fall.

As an African American woman, I am acutely aware that my vagina and myself are perceived as "different" from other owners of vaginas. My vagina is "angry." It is an overtly sexual place, not a sacred one. My vagina is the one you fuck and leave, or fuck and impregnate and leave—impregnation being the more desirable outcome—not the one you marry and show off in wedding photos. My vagina is hidden, hungry, deviant, voracious, dangerous, delinquent, domineering, and must be tamed, much like my very self. From where do these notions arise?

Unfortunately, like most other systemically ingrained opinions on race, these deep-seated beliefs about the difference between White and Black vaginas likely come from the 19th century. White vaginas were timid and fragile, and White women were seen as delicate, sensitive, and "frigid." White vaginas needed to be coaxed into sexual activity. Conversely, Black vaginas were hypersexual and lascivious, mindlessly craving sex, and these beliefs not only persist today but are likely worse than they have ever been, given the advent of the internet and social media. One particular historical culprit we can target for starting this is Dr. J. Marion Sims and his camp. Sims was a slave owner, physician, and shameless self-promoter who became infamous for his work on the vaginas of enslaved females and the beliefs he and those like him have perpetuated generations later.

J. MARION SIMS, FATHER OF RACIST VAGINALISM

During the time of Dr. J. Marion Sims, enslaved women were seen not only as workers, but also as breeders. Their vaginas were routinely raped by their owners to satisfy the rapists' appetites for sex and power. Of course, this also gave rapists the benefit of making more slave children. This is where the "one drop = Black" rule originated; it stemmed from an early law (1662) regarding children born of Black women and White men: Those children were slaves. This way, even the mixed-race humans could be slaves and make money for the masters. In addition, if an enslaved woman did have a husband or partner with whom to form a family unit, he was often either sold away or forced to impregnate other enslaved women, weakening the bonds between husband and wife.

This early access of male owners to "easy" sex via rape and the devaluation of Black women to their physical attributes is what stifles us to this very day, resulting in our modern-day perception of Black women as sexualized and soulless. Given how there was a clear impetus to keep enslaved women working and their vaginas producing more slaves, those women who suffered a vaginal trauma or fistula from birth injuries or repeated rape were considered "useless." Although the women could still work, given the leakage of urine and/or stool, they were sexually (and thus reproductively) undesirable.

Enter Sims. He was a general practice doctor in Montgomery, Alabama, in the 19th century. The population of Montgomery at that time was two-thirds Black, and as a general physician, Sims would have seen any case brought by White slave owners given his need for business. Even though in his own words he stated, "If there was anything I hated, it was investigating the organs of the female pelvis," he somehow became a primary referral doctor for vesicovaginal fistula, primarily through barbaric surgical trials on enslaved women.[1]

The Sims family did hold ownership of humans, and as his biography details, it was another slave owner who brought him his first fistula case, a lady named Anarcha. We only have first names for the patients who were named at all. Any other personal information about these ladies has been utterly lost to history, leaving us to only deduce insights about them. What we do know is that after enduring a difficult birth with a forceps delivery, Anarcha was found to have developed a fistula and was brought back to Sims, who had performed the delivery. Because Sims "hated" gynecology, he sent her back to the plantation without treatment.

Sometime later, a White woman who had been thrown from a horse and sustained some trauma to her pelvis was brought in. As we now know, early physicians thought the uterus was prone to wandering off and needed to be put back; Sims assumed the same with this patient and sought to find her lost uterus. This is when he realized, after putting the patient in the knee-to-chest position and inserting two fingers, that he could actually see inside the vagina and may have the possibility of seeing a fistula enough to repair it.

This discovery of adequate visualization led him to examine another enslaved woman, Lucy, who was brought to his makeshift backyard hospital to see if he could repair her fistula. He found he could use a bent spoon (yes, an actual spoon) to see inside. This led to the development of the Sims speculum. (While most websites credit him with the invention of the modern speculum, I would like to reiterate that it was actually a French woman, Madame Marie Anne Boivin, who came up with the self-retaining speculum concept that we now know and hate.)

Over the course of years, he performed multiple surgeries on enslaved women suffering from fistula, trying and failing to remedy the situation. Lucy once had a sponge left inside her and nearly died of infection. She did not perish and lived to get operated on many more times. There were three women in particular featured in his writings: Lucy, Anarcha, and Betsy. Despite the belief that slave women were not fully human and of subpar intelligence, he trained them all to be surgical assistants during each other's surgeries. These were all done without the benefit of any type of anesthesia or pain control. I cannot imagine the complete and utter anguish they all endured over the years, and being made to help time and time again with the knowledge that the surgery might not work must have made it just that much more difficult.

FIG. 15.1

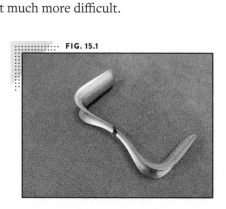

SIMS'S SPECULUM. YOU CAN STILL FIND THESE IN SURGICAL TRAYS TODAY.

Why was this OK? Well, dear reader, you are probably chalking this up to slavery being a dark period when horrible things happened, and you are correct, to a certain degree. But the reason such horrors were carried out was a sense (that persists today) of Black women being "other"—alien, dark, different, and not quite human—making it easier to objectify them and use them for experimentation. I might even argue that the beginnings of the "strong Black woman" myth originated during this time and was bolstered by Dr. Sims's writings. The same argument of "otherizing" was made by the Germans about their "other": Jews during the Holocaust. Making someone appear to be less than human allows other humans to do the most inhumane things.

Say their names: Lucy, Anarcha, Betsy.

They deserve to be remembered.

VAGINA DENTATA MYTHS AS AN ORIGIN OF RAPE CULTURE

The subjugation and brutalization of women has been justified throughout history with many tales and myths. One of the more interesting is that of the *vagina dentata*, or the "toothed vagina." The story is similar throughout many ancient cultures, all of which involve vaginas having teeth and some type of violence to the vagina to remove them. In fact, there are variations on this theme in Native American, Asian, Middle Eastern, Christian, Polynesian, and South American cultures, crossing all continents.

The female genitalia was (and still is) seen as a mysterious chasm, a dark place where men lose themselves in the "little death" of orgasm. The Greeks even believed that as a man ejaculated, he lost some of his vital life force, and the woman would "eat" it up, since the Greek word *sema* (where we get "semen") meant both "seed" and "food." As an English major, it was my job to research and attempt to draw conclusions in a coherent way about all manner of topics and to support my argument appropriately. Therefore, let us look at these varying myths and how they relate to today and allow me to support a theory: The myth of the vagina dentata relates not only to Freud's castration anxiety theory, but to present-day misogyny. We shall start with one particular short story from central India, documented in the *British Medical Journal* in 1943:

> *A Brahmin and his very beautiful daughter came to a Baiga's house to beg. After they had been fed, the Brahmin lay down to sleep, and the girl went into the garden to steal some cucumbers for their supper. The Baiga caught her in the field and raped her. But she had teeth in her vagina and with these she cut off the Baiga's penis. He began to shout with pain. His elder brother's wife, who was in love with him, had been watching to see if he would go to see the Brahmin girl or not, and when she heard the noise she ran to the field and said to the girl, "Put back the bit you have cut off, or I'll tell your father." At that the girl was frightened and she put the penis back in its place. When it was fixed on again, the Baiga lay the girl down and pulled out the teeth with a bit of string. The Baiga soon found himself in love with the Brahmin girl, and they ran off together to get married.*[2]

The idea of vagina as maneater exists in other cultures in slightly different ways. Take this myth from the Sioux. There was a beautiful and seductive woman who accepted the love of a young warrior. They went into a cloud to be together (sexually). When the cloud disappeared, the warrior was gone, with only bones remaining, snakes slithering and gnawing at his bones. The seductress literally ate him.

A Hawaiian myth tells of another story of vaginas behaving badly. The demi-god Maui desired to cheat death. Maui's father told him of one of his ancestors, a goddess of night and death named Hine-nui-te-pō. Maui decided he would enter her (through her vagina, of course), cut out her heart, and emerge victoriously through her mouth. Going in the way he came out (from a vaginal birth) was supposed to reverse the process of death. So he gave it a try. Changing into an eel, he made his way into her vagina. Unfortunately, even though the first mouth didn't get him, the second one (the real one) did, and he was cut in half. So ends Maui, eaten by a powerful woman. He does live on in the name of a beautiful island in the Pacific, though.[3]

Most vagina dentata myths tend to follow the same construct. Beautiful girl has teeth in vagina. Girl injures man's penis through coitus, although rape is the more common story. Girl has to have teeth removed, usually through some violent means. Girl and (more often than not) rapist live happily ever after. Consider the reasons behind these myths, which involve some sort of a severe "taming of the shrew," if you will. Each of these derivations give us a beautiful yet headstrong or disobedient woman who must somehow be subdued in order to find happiness in a heterosexual marriage or relationship. It also reinforces to men the dangers inherent in a beautiful woman, that she may literally bite off your penis and consume you, leaving you with nothing.

The idea of vagina as a mouth full of dangerous, biting teeth may contribute to the idea that rape is allowable if it is a means to an end. That end being to save the man from figurative castration, the Freudian, psychological kind, saving him from being subjugated or pussy-whipped by a dangerous woman. These subtle, perhaps even subliminal, messages that have worked their way from ancient times to the present may be one of the sources of misogyny and perhaps even the rape culture we have to deal with today. Why do I say that? Well, take this messaging, for example. Look at movies like *Alien* (1979), *Predator* (1987), and *Starship Troopers* (1997). Each of these films features a horrible vagina-monster as its villain. Each of these monsters is subdued by hypermasculine men (or a large phallus, if you're talking about *Alien*).

Therefore, if men can place women into a different category than themselves, characterizing them as monstrous, deviant, and deadly, it's easier for men to justify their fear and insecurity manifested as hatred, believing that they must somehow "knock out her teeth" and render her helpless and willing to have sex. While in India, where the most common of the vagina dentata myths originate, a rape is reported once every fifteen minutes, don't think that we here in the US get off easy. A hate group of men called Incels, short for involuntary celibates, emerged during the 2010s. Because vaginas are perceived to be dark and dangerous, they believe they need to "tame" them, perhaps violently, even to the point of death. And they have done so. Incel attacks in Canada (Canada, no less!) have killed more than two dozen people. And with the reach of the internet, this number is unfortunately poised to grow as these entitled men seek to assert their belief that they deserve sex. This of course is the dumbest thing ever, but we can take solace in the fact that if one of them goes to jail after committing one of these heinous acts, the sex they'll be getting certainly won't be what they're looking for.[4]

Conversely, the movie *Teeth* is a prime example of "pussy grabs back." This 2008 movie takes a different view of the vagina dentata. It does not involve the vagina's teeth being forcibly removed and the assaulted woman and her assailant riding off into the sunset in marriage. Instead, the main character, a young woman named Dawn (a spokesperson for the community's local chastity group, no less), is raped. As a result of this assault, she develops teeth, and well, let the hijinks begin. Apparently, Dawn's super vagina can tell the difference between an honorable boy and one whose motives are not quite so sincere. Sounds like a rather nice gift to have, no? As penises pile up, Dawn begins to realize her special feminine power and becomes something of a vagina vigilante. One review of the movie reads as such: "We haven't had a good vagina dentata movie in theaters lately, so it's a pleasure to see *Teeth* filling that particular need with such obvious relish and style."[5]

While a biting vagina may make for comedy gold, my question is, why do we need a vagina dentata movie in the first place? Does perpetuating myths through movies such as this help or hurt the vagina-wielding population? Given that popular culture still makes the vagina seem dangerous and dark, I shout no. Vaginas get enough of a bad rap.[6]

And speaking of rap, as I was working on this chapter, something made me think back to the cover of one of my favorite albums from the 1990s.

Was that a vagina dentata on their album cover? I looked, and yes it was. The Pharcyde was (is?) an edgy and snarky hip-hop/rap group whose lyrics were almost as biting as their cover. Now I wonder, how many who purchased this album understood the symbolism? Can we somehow interpret this rendering as a positive, or as you look at the characters, do we understand their fear, resignation, or excitement at being devoured by the ultimate vagina dentata?

THE FEW ACTUAL MEDICAL DIFFERENCES BETWEEN VAGINAS

Of course, researching anthropologic and morphologic differences between ethnic groups is a sensitive subject and is quite difficult to address objectively. During my search, I only found a very few studies that examined the specific shape of the vagina and how it may vary between groups, and in fact, most of the studies came from the same research group, so there may be some inherent bias here. In one study from 2000, researchers, in order to determine the shape of the vagina, used the same stuff dentists use to make casts of your teeth to make vaginal casts. Not sure how they got it out after hardening was complete; I can't imagine it was pleasant. Vaginas don't open wide like mouths can unless there's a baby involved.

In their study, they examined twenty-three African American, thirty-nine Caucasian, and fifteen Latina women in three positions: lying, sitting, and standing. What they discovered was interesting. They discovered another archetypal vagina shape to add to those previously known: the pumpkin seed (see the image from chapter 1), which was noted in 40 percent of the African American women. This shape is narrower at the introitus and again at the top of the vagina near the cervix. For Latina vaginas, they found the heart shape to be the most prevalent, narrow at the introitus and roomier at the top. The various shapes—parallel, slug, conical, and heart—had been elucidated in a previous paper and were distributed relatively equally among Whites, who were the first group studied. However, after gathering these new data, they discovered the overall introital measurements of African Americans to be smaller than that of other groups. Keep in mind this is the only study like this done to date, and it was a small one at that. I would hazard to say that we would probably see a clearer, more complete picture if we had a larger study population, and of course included more ethnicities and body types. Unfortunately, there probably aren't a lot of researchers interested in this particular topic so we have to learn what we can from the information we have. It appears to me that the overarching theme is that vaginas vary.[7]

These racial vagina differences may have clinical implications. We learned about how sometimes the uterus, bladder, and even rectum can herniate through the vagina and cause all sorts of trouble. We have learned that in many cases, some vaginas are more resilient than others when it comes to prolapse. Data suggest that African American women have a lower prevalence of symptomatic pelvic organ prolapse than other racial or ethnic groups. A study of more than 2,200 women bears this out. The researchers found that the risk in Latina and White women had a four- to five-fold increased risk of prolapse when compared to African American women. While it is not certain exactly why that is, it might be the vaginal shape that contributes to this. Since it appears that the pumpkin seed–shaped vagina is more common in African American women, a narrower vaginal introitus (opening) may keep the pelvic organs from falling out.[8]

There are some differences between the shape of pelvises (hips), too. We've known this for quite some time, and you probably have seen it yourself given the number of music videos focused on bottoms, with some women having naturally curvy bottoms and some others spending money to get them. Apparently, this shape has always been of fascination, starting all the way back with the "Hottentot Venus."

Saartjie Bartmann was born in what is now known as South Africa in 1789 as a member of the Khoikhoi people—Hottentot is a derogatory term made up by the Dutch for the native people of this area. She was not enslaved, but many an unfortunate event befell this young woman. Her mother died when she was very young, and both her father and fiancé were killed during a European ambush at her engagement party. She was just a teenager at the time. She was exploited by a man named Hendrik Caesars, a black South African in whose house she took work (which shows that Black people not sticking together goes way back).[9]

Caesars introduced her to Alexander Dunlop, a British military doctor who was fascinated by her naturally occurring body shape, complete with a round, shapely bottom. She was then taken to England where her backside was put on nearly full display. They dressed her in a ridiculous outfit that included a skin-tight flesh-colored catsuit, headdress, beads, a spear, and a pipe.

Her body type, now known to be completely normal, was seen as an aberration, a freakshow, and it didn't help that the fashion of the day had already begun to emphasize the backside. While Englishwomen had to put extra cloth there to achieve the shape they desired, here was a woman who had it all on her own. Perhaps there was jealousy mixed in with the fascination? In addition, Lord Granville, a well-known member of the British Parliament at the time, who was rumored to want to take over after the King, had an equally impressive derriere. The media of the day had quite a time comparing the two.

After abolitionists in England lobbied for Bartmann's freedom, she was moved to France and continued to be exhibited. Unfortunately, the French treated her no better, and Bartmann died at the age of 26, possibly of pneumonia. This is where more seeds of racist vaginalism were solidified. After her death, her body became even more of a spectacle, and despite the fact that she spoke English, Dutch, and some French, her intelligence was compared to that of an orangutan, of course because of her protuberant bottom. Additionally, the "scientists" examining her were also quite interested in why her labia were enlarged (again, we know this is normal). Her brain, buttocks, and genitals were preserved, and a plaster cast was made of her body and displayed in the Musée d'Homme in France until—wait for it—1976. She was finally returned home to South Africa in 2002. What this illustrates for us is that normal variations in anatomy, vaginas included, have been used to justify racist vaginalism since antiquity, and they should be considered with caution in all scenarios.[10]

FIG. 15.2

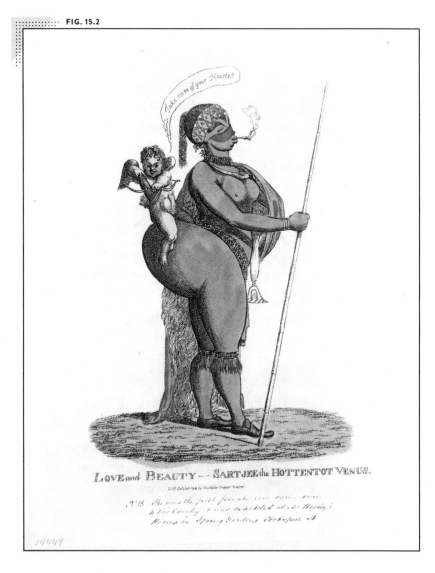

A DRAWING OF THE "HOTTENTOT VENUS," A CARICATURE DRESSED IN OUTLANDISH GARB INDICATIVE OF NO KNOWN NATIVE DRESS.

Of course, hips and body types vary widely. While more of an academic exercise than a regular obstetric practice, "clinical pelvimetry," or measuring the pelvis, first with X-ray and now with MRI, can tell you exactly how your pelvis is shaped. These shapes will certainly vary between ethnicities as individual genetics plays just as great a role as population genetics. Of course, it's not like if you have this measurement taken or if you are of this or that ethnic group, we tell you that you MUST have a C-section and can't deliver your kid the regular way, through your vagina. But because we're talking about race and vagina differences, I believe this to be a relevant discussion.

FIG. 15.3

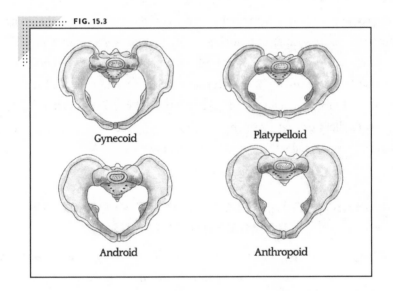

Gynecoid

Platypelloid

Android

Anthropoid

THE FOUR GENERAL TYPES OF PELVISES.

The so-called "most favorable pelvis type for a vaginal birth" is the gynecoid type. This is considered the classic female shape, with hips as wide as shoulders, with some butt to the back. I say "hips and booty."

The android pelvic type is a narrow pelvis, somewhat more similar to that of a male. Shoulders are wider than hips, and it is known that labor can be more, well, laborious, as a baby has a harder time moving through the smaller space. Many women with this pelvis may need a cesarean section, depending on the size of the baby, but we still recommend laboring for a vaginal birth. Not much hips or booty here.

Anthropoid pelvises are another variation on the female pelvis. While the hip part is not so wide, the front to back space is ample. So while shoulders are wider than hips, there's plenty of business in the back, and it is generally spacious enough for a vaginal delivery. This is my pelvis shape, by the way. No hips, but booty, often somewhat more to the back than a gynecoid. Ms. Bartmann's pelvis was likely a gynecoid/anthropoid amalgamation, with both ample hips and, of course, booty.

Platypelloid pelvises are wide, and these women have the classic hourglass figure—hips, but no booty—with hips sometimes wider than shoulders. Unfortunately, they don't have much business in the back. Some of these ladies have trouble delivering vaginally because the pelvic opening is flat. But if you believe you have this type, don't be dismayed. Modern obstetrics dictates that everyone, barring some exceptions, will be given a chance to bring a baby through the vagina/pelvis.[10]

BIAS AND DEVELOPMENT OF VAGINALISM IN MODERN CULTURE

When we refer to vaginalism, we are all affected in one way or another, judging ourselves and each other into oblivion. How do these perceived White and Black vaginalisms manifest in real women's lives today? While White and Black women alike are afflicted by anxiety and depression from being subjugated for centuries, Black women deal with the added indignity of no one seeming to care or even believe we are in pain. So when we present with symptoms of anxiety, depression, or pain, we receive a different diagnosis from White women. Why? Vaginalisms that have developed throughout the centuries have solidified our otherness into easy to quantify categories and thus explain away our very humanity.

Pain perception

Historically speaking, Black women have always been characterized as the bearers of pain. From Lucy, Anarcha, and Betsy's "stoic" bearing of pain while enduring Sims's tortuous surgeries to my own patients' experiences, the myth that Black women either do not feel pain like others or are better at "taking" pain is pervasive.[11]

Take a particular condition called endometriosis. Endometriosis is a painful affliction of the female pelvis that theoretically develops when endometrial tissue implants in the pelvis through the fallopian tubes instead of leaving the body through the vagina during menstruation. Each month, and oftentimes throughout the month, this tissue is activated by hormonal cues and can cause symptoms ranging from mild cramping to debilitating pain, nausea, and gastrointestinal and bladder symptoms. Historically, endometriosis has been seen as a condition of the upper-middle-class woman who has delayed childbearing, with this clogging of the tubes a result of waiting too long, resulting in infertility. This belief has been debunked, of course, as endometriosis can start to take hold in a woman's early twenties. Additionally, bear in mind there has been no epidemiological difference between any racial or ethnic groups with regard to the prevalence of endometriosis. However, as late as 2019, analysis of several studies show that endometriosis continues to be underdiagnosed in African American women, and diagnosed more often in Whites and Asians. It seems Black women's complaints of pain go untreated, undertreated, or outright ignored.

I wish I had a snarky comment to make about this to lighten the mood, but unfortunately this is just not to be. So if Black women show up in pain with the same pattern as Whites and other groups, what is their diagnosis? Well, take a wild guess.

They are diagnosed with having had an STD.

When Black women show up to a physician's office or emergency department with pain similar to that of endometriosis, they are diagnosed more often with a condition called pelvic inflammatory disease (PID).

PID is an inflammation of the pelvis that stems from having had a bout of gonorrhea or chlamydia sometime in your life, and it can lead to painful episodes, scarring, and, like endometriosis, infertility.

Black women have been fighting to be seen as pain-feeling humans for decades. One of my old mentors, Dr. Donald Chatman, wrote about this in 1976, when I was a mere one-year-old. Dr. Chatman was a well-known and well-respected gynecologist and academician of his day and the first Black president of the American Association of Gynecologic Laparoscopists. Because the definitive diagnosis of endometriosis is made with laparoscopic surgery, he took a look at many patients. What he discovered is what we are still writing about today, half a lifetime later. He discovered that more than 20 percent of African American women diagnosed with pelvic inflammatory disease actually had endometriosis. Meaning, we were being treated for STDs we didn't have, just because of the color of our vaginas.[12]

Although the idea that Black women are better at taking pain had its roots in slavery, this thinking continues to this very day. On more than one occasion, I have had to tell my resident physicians and students that making an incision on a black vagina is just the same as on a White one—Black skin is not "thicker" or "tougher" to cut than anyone else's.[13] Before a surgery, I'm usually the one to cover my African American patient's breasts as she lays nude while being positioned for surgery, when my other patients are magically blanketed. When my patients are being sent home, I've often had to double-check to make sure my Black patients are sent home with enough medication to manage their pain after surgery. I've had those very same patients tell me that they felt "rushed" out of the hospital after surgery and that their pain needs were not addressed.

According to a study from the *American Journal of Emergency Medicine* in 2019, African American patients were 40 percent less likely to receive medication when compared to White patients, and 34 percent less likely to be given opioids for pain relief.[14] One of the main reasons that African Americans have been largely spared the horror of the opioid epidemic is because we were not prescribed pain management to the same extent as

Whites. A blessing in disguise. It is the rare occasion that I have a White patient complain of a lack of pain control while in the hospital after surgery. And the fact that I am sitting on my sofa in 2020 writing about this is not lost upon me. Although bias in medicine is becoming a hot topic as of late, we have a long way to go before we are anywhere close to reaching parity. But at least knowledge of our own biases and the production of more academic literature is a good first step. And you, dear patient, must help us by leading the way, whether you have a Black, Latina, White, or Asian vagina. We with vaginas must unite.

Insist that you be heard.

Enlist the help of others.

Persist in your concerns.

THE ANGRY BLACK WOMAN, THE WHORE, AND THE MAMMY

Why are Black women's vaginas seen as overtly sexual and little black girls' vaginas seen as more mature? I think you already know where I am going with this. Black women, when it comes to honorable desirability, always seem to cling to the lowest rung on the ladder, saddled with hundreds of years of societal manipulation and suppression. Other vaginas may benefit from their perceived qualities—White vaginas are seen as delicate, Asian vaginas as submissive, and Latina vaginas as saucy and sassy. These images are generally positive, desirable, and acceptable. In contrast, we as Black women have the difficulty of having to walk the tightrope at every turn. If we rightfully assert ourselves when the situation calls, we are the Angry Black Woman. If we explore our natural sexuality, we are the Whore, the Jezebel. If we show our nurturing side, then we are a Mammy. My question is, when we as Black women find a way to capitalize on these stereotypical misconceptions, are we helping or hurting ourselves? Or is it simply the only way we have left to survive? Allow me to explore these caricatures: the Angry Black Woman, the Whore, and the Mammy.

Sapphire, the "Angry Black Woman"

First is the Sapphire character, otherwise known as the Angry Black Woman. You are absolutely forgiven if you do not know where the name Sapphire came from; I had to discover it myself during this research. In 1928, the *Amos 'n' Andy* show aired on CBS radio, beginning as a sort of minstrel show, with White men vocalizing the silly and inept black characters. In the show, Amos and Andy were members of a fictional Black fraternal order, and one of the characters, George "Kingfish" Stephens, had a particularly acrid wife whose name was Sapphire. Mr. Stephens's character represented the worst of what America thought of Black men—a lazy, broke, unredeemable, get-rich-quick schemer—and Sapphire took great pleasure in castigating and emasculating him for his shortcomings.

Examples of the Sapphire Angry Black Woman only increase exponentially from those early beginnings. You're already thinking of them right now. Although the quintessential 21st-century ABW is Omarosa Manigault Newman (although she needs only one name), she is hardly the only one; this is merely a result of decades of development. Think back to shows like *Good Times*, *The Jeffersons*, and even *Martin*. Each of these featured a loud-mouthed African American woman blaming and berating not only Black men, but everyone in her neighborhood. Even I myself was branded the ABW during my brief fifteen minutes of fame while on the reality show *The Mole*, primarily due to careful editing. Thank goodness I get to live that down because the show wasn't that popular. The question is: Can we blame Omarosa and those before her for capitalizing on the caricature? It is not my place to say, having been a victim of it myself. But the result is that any African American woman who even begins to speak up for herself or others is automatically branded as "angry."

This is evident by the words of Cal Thomas, a commentator for Fox Television:

> *Look at the image of angry black women on television. Politically you have Maxine Waters of California, liberal Democrat.*

She's always angry every time she gets on television. Cynthia McKinney, another angry black woman. And who are the black women you see on the local news at night in cities all over the country. They're usually angry about something. They've had a son who has been shot in a drive-by shooting. They are angry at Bush. So you don't really have a profile of non-angry black women, of whom there are quite a few.[15]

Thomas, admittedly not a trained sociologist, expressed what many Americans see and internalize, namely, images of Sapphires: angry at Black men, White men, White women, the federal government, racism, maybe life itself. Thomas, shortly after making his statements about Black women, agreed with a co-panelist that Oprah Winfrey is one of the not-angry ones.

No matter how articulate we are, whenever we speak up or express our rights to an opinion, we are branded as Sapphires. Even our own beloved Michelle Obama was not exempt. At the beginning of the Obamas' rise, she was difficult to categorize. Here was a Harvard-educated woman, a mother, an attorney, who having grown up on the South Side of Chicago was smart enough to know how scrutinized she would be. She "went high" at every turn, threading the needle, avoiding being typed as Mammy, Jezebel, or Sapphire. Until one day she mentioned how, "for the first time in my adult life I am proud of my country because it feels like hope is finally making a comeback."[16] It was then she was branded as the Sapphire, the angry Black woman. For expressing pride in her country.

While we will later discover why the Fox commentators agreed that Ms. Winfrey is not angry, it is clear that the Sapphire stereotype has permeated as the dominant societal view of African American vaginas. Even for the venerable Mrs. Michelle Obama.

The Jezebel, the "Whore"

The next moniker African American women have been saddled with is the Jezebel, the whore. This is the hypersexual, seductive temptress, the maneater (toothed vagina, anyone?) who exploits weak men through her sexuality. The European fascination with the societal customs of some African continental tribes, such as polygamy and the physical anatomy of those on the continent (remember our Hottentot Venus), contributed to this image from the 17th century onward. The Jezebel character was also developed as a patsy for White slaveowners' lust, allowing them to blame the woman for their own indiscretions. Over the years, the concept of the Jezebel morphed from plantation whore of the 1800s to welfare queen of the 1980s. In 1978, President Ronald Reagan stoked the fears of the public by speaking at length about a supposed "welfare queen" in Chicago who was rumored to be living high on the hog off the government, having defrauded various government entities of hundreds of thousands of dollars.[17] She also popped out children at her leisure, leaving several befuddled husbands in her wake. While Reagan insinuated that this supposed queen was Black, allowing people to assume what they would, the real person he was referring to was listed in the 1930 census as White, as was her entire family. However, this simple omission galvanized an entire movement against supposed welfare fraud perpetrated by Jezebel African American women that persists today.

Often combined with the Sapphire persona, some of the most well-known examples of the Jezebel in popular culture are the characters in the Blaxploitation films of the 1970s, during what I call the Pimps and Hoes period. These sex workers, or Hoes, appeared to be superheroes, with beautiful sexy bodies, pulling guns out from only God knows where for the good of all, but they actually played into the stereotype of the powerful, remorseless, dangerous temptress. You can't imagine a movie in an urban setting without having the stereotypical Black whore on the streets. Again, can we fault actresses such as the phenomenal Pam Grier or Halle Berry for taking the acting work given to them, even though they had to play these kinds of characters? While there was plenty of criticism for Berry's movie *Monster's Ball*, it garnered her an Oscar. Now, we could certainly debate why this particular role was the one that deserved that award. This is especially irksome given the movie's plot that harkens back to the practical arrangements many enslaved women made with their White captors, paired with Berry's character's lewdness and lack of education. These portrayals only harden the ingrained stereotypes that have emerged over hundreds of years.

The adultification, which means that small children are treated as being more mature, including having innate knowledge of sex, of Black girls' vaginas also falls into the Jezebel category, peppered with a little Sapphire. Due to the vestigial views from slavery that little girls were simply breeders in waiting, Black girls suffer disproportionately from adultification. A study from the Center on Poverty and Inequality from Georgetown Law revealed that adultification and its many pitfalls are real. Black girls were more likely to be disciplined for talking back (being a Sapphire). They were also seen as needing less nurturing and help than equivocal White counterparts. The study looked at age groups from 0 to 16 and discovered these views started much earlier than one might expect, well before puberty: "That is, beginning as early as 5 years of age, Black girls were more likely to be viewed as behaving and seeming older than their stated age; more knowledgeable about adult topics, including sex; and more likely to take on adult roles and responsibilities than what would have been expected for their age."[18]

While little Black girls' vaginas suffer from the vestiges of slavery, the African American woman as Jezebel whore is now being used by women themselves to further their own gains. We now knowingly hoist racist vaginalism upon ourselves for the sake of social media followers, views, downloads, and the like, while not acknowledging the double standard that exists between vaginas of different shades and cultures. For example, we look at outrageous stars such as Madonna or Lady Gaga as empowering, while artists such as Nicki Minaj and Megan Thee Stallion have been put down as whores. While both groups use their bodies as sexual conduits, it is only the Black vaginas that get scrutinized as Jezebels. While many academics debate the quandary of those Black women, especially those who seek fame by utilizing their femininity and sexuality, it is not my place to criticize these women. My only goal is to bring it to your attention as a vagina-wielding human so you can become aware and combat it by seeing it as what it is: a double standard. The next time you read about or see different vagina owners behaving in a similar way but getting different responses from the mainstream, consider this.

Mammy, the "Nurturing Asexual"

The first Mammy one may think of is the most infamous one, played by Hattie McDaniel in *Gone With the Wind*. She was a pleasantly plump, expressively supportive slave woman in Scarlett O'Hara's family home. McDaniel got an Oscar for this portrayal (are we sensing a pattern?). Historians now reveal to us that the Mammy caricature probably didn't exist during slavery. To allow an enslaved person to be able to eat so much as to become chubby AND live to be in middle age was rare at best. Those we refer to as "house slaves" such as the Mammy were probably fair-skinned teenagers, likely quite skinny. The prevailing thought now is that Mammy-ism and its associations were probably developed after Reconstruction to convince the dominant society that slavery wasn't that bad, that people enjoyed living and serving for free, and to reinforce the caste system and hierarchy. While Mammy began as a stereotype, she morphed into a powerful and enduring symbol of the romantic, slave-owning South, a myth that haunts Black vaginas to this day.[19]

Our current society is not exempt. While the use of the Mammy stereotype has evolved somewhat from *Gone With the Wind*, it has yet to disappear completely. Here are a few examples of media that capitalizes on the Mammy stereotype:

Gimme a Break

The Help

Aunt Jemima

Oprah

Why does Oprah have no White equal? Why is it that there is no chubby, friendly White woman helping you live your best life? The reason harkens right back to the discussion at hand. Unfortunately, the likely reason is that Oprah equates to the Mammy culture.[20]

Oprah is friendly, fat, and asexual. She placates White women, just like Mammies were thought to have done during slavery. She's happy and helpful. Although Mammies allegedly cooked, cleaned, and helped raise children (not her own), instead Oprah now helps you "live your best life," never having had her own children. The verbiage has changed, but the truth lies beneath. Now I think it quite phenomenal that this woman has been able to accomplish what she has, becoming a billionaire and all, and even though she will NEVER admit that she has used her own stereotype as a Black Mammy figure to achieve massive financial gain, she knows. Just like Minaj and her voluminous bottom, she has used known stereotypes to make gains at the expense of the whole. But don't worry Oprah, I'll keep your secret.[21]

Vaginalisms are prevalent and pervasive; we've been living with them for far too long. Unfortunately, we as women tend to play into our assigned roles, occasionally for personal gain but mainly for survival. It is only when we keep all -isms (sexism, feminism, racism) in mind, every day, whether it be for your vagina or someone else's, that vaginalisms will become merely vaginas, and we will have overcome. Let us not vajayjay; let us vagina.

> **DID YOU KNOW?**
>
> The first Black female ob-gyn was Dr. Helen Octavia Dickens, who attended the University of Illinois (my alma mater) and received board certification in 1945. This chapter was for you. Given what I endured, I can only imagine how you endured.

Female Sexual Function Index (FSFI)

NSTRUCTIONS: These questions ask about your sexual feelings and responses during the past four weeks. Please answer the following questions as honestly and clearly as possible. Your responses will be kept completely confidential. In answering these questions, the following definitions apply:

Sexual activity can include caressing, foreplay, masturbation, and vaginal intercourse.

Sexual intercourse is defined as penile penetration (entry) of the vagina.

Sexual stimulation includes situations like foreplay with a partner, self-stimulation (masturbation), or sexual fantasy.

Circle one response per question.

1. Over the past four weeks, how often did you feel sexual desire or interest?

   5 = Almost always or always
   4 = Most times (more than half the time)
   3 = Sometimes (about half the time)
   2 = A few times (less than half the time)
   1 = Almost never or never

2. Over the past four weeks, how would you rate your level (degree) of sexual desire or interest?

5 = Very high
4 = High
3 = Moderate
2 = Low
1 = Very low or none at all

3. Over the past four weeks, how often did you feel sexually aroused ("turned on") during sexual activity or intercourse?

0 = No sexual activity
5 = Almost always or always
4 = Most times (more than half the time)
3 = Sometimes (about half the time)
2 = A few times (less than half the time)
1 = Almost never or never

4. Over the past four weeks, how would you rate your level of sexual arousal ("turn on") during sexual activity or intercourse?

0 = No sexual activity
5 = Very high
4 = High
3 = Moderate
2 = Low
1 = Very low or none at all

5. Over the past four weeks, how confident were you about becoming sexually aroused during sexual activity or intercourse?

0 = No sexual activity
5 = Very high confidence

4 = High confidence

3 = Moderate confidence

2 = Low confidence

1 = Very low or no confidence

6. Over the past four weeks, how often have you been satisfied with your arousal (excitement) during sexual activity or intercourse?

0 = No sexual activity

5 = Almost always or always

4 = Most times (more than half the time)

3 = Sometimes (about half the time)

2 = A few times (less than half the time)

1 = Almost never or never

7. Over the past four weeks, how often did you become lubricated ("wet") during sexual activity or intercourse?

0 = No sexual activity

5 = Almost always or always

4 = Most times (more than half the time)

3 = Sometimes (about half the time)

2 = A few times (less than half the time)

1 = Almost never or never

8. Over the past four weeks, how difficult was it to become lubricated ("wet") during sexual activity or intercourse?

0 = No sexual activity

1 = Extremely difficult or impossible

2 = Very difficult

3 = Difficult

4 = Slightly difficult

5 = Not difficult

9. Over the past four weeks, how often did you maintain your lubrication ("wetness") until completion of sexual activity or intercourse?

0 = No sexual activity

5 = Almost always or always

4 = Most times (more than half the time)

3 = Sometimes (about half the time)

2 = A few times (less than half the time)

1 = Almost never or never

10. Over the past four weeks, how difficult was it to maintain your lubrication ("wetness") until completion of sexual activity or intercourse?

0 = No sexual activity

1 = Extremely difficult or impossible

2 = Very difficult

3 = Difficult

4 = Slightly difficult

5 = Not difficult

11. Over the past four weeks, when you had sexual stimulation or intercourse, how often did you reach orgasm (climax)?

0 = No sexual activity

5 = Almost always or always

4 = Most times (more than half the time)

3 = Sometimes (about half the time)

2 = A few times (less than half the time)

1 = Almost never or never

12. Over the past four weeks, when you had sexual stimulation or intercourse, how difficult was it for you to reach orgasm (climax)?

0 = No sexual activity

1 = Extremely difficult or impossible

2 = Very difficult

3 = Difficult

4 = Slightly difficult

5 = Not difficult

13. Over the past four weeks, how satisfied were you with your ability to reach orgasm (climax) during sexual activity or intercourse?

0 = No sexual activity

5 = Very satisfied

4 = Moderately satisfied

3 = About equally satisfied and dissatisfied

2 = Moderately dissatisfied

1 = Very dissatisfied

14. Over the past four weeks, how satisfied have you been with the amount of emotional closeness during sexual activity between you and your partner?

0 = No sexual activity

5 = Very satisfied

4 = Moderately satisfied

3 = About equally satisfied and dissatisfied

2 = Moderately dissatisfied

1 = Very dissatisfied

15. Over the past four weeks, how satisfied have you been with your sexual relationship with your partner?

5 = Very satisfied

4 = Moderately satisfied

3 = About equally satisfied and dissatisfied

2 = Moderately dissatisfied

1 = Very dissatisfied

16. Over the past four weeks, how satisfied have you been with your overall sexual life?

5 = Very satisfied

4 = Moderately satisfied

3 = About equally satisfied and dissatisfied

2 = Moderately dissatisfied

1 = Very dissatisfied

17. Over the past four weeks, how often did you experience discomfort or pain during vaginal penetration?

0 = Did not attempt intercourse

1 = Almost always or always

2 = Most times (more than half the time)

3 = Sometimes (about half the time)

4 = A few times (less than half the time)

5 = Almost never or never

18. Over the past four weeks, how often did you experience discomfort or pain following vaginal penetration?

0 = Did not attempt intercourse

1 = Almost always or always

2 = Most times (more than half the time)

3 = Sometimes (about half the time)

4 = A few times (less than half the time)

5 = Almost never or never

19. Over the past four weeks, how would you rate your level (degree) of discomfort or pain during or following vaginal penetration?

0 = Did not attempt intercourse

1 = Very high

2 = High

3 = Moderate

4 = Low

5 = Very low or none at all

Higher scores indicate lesser difficulty and more satisfaction with sex. If you find your score on the low end, please see your practitioner. Thanks to www.fsfiquestionnaire.com

Appendix B

Amazing Sex Toys,

chosen by Searah Desaych of Early 2 Bed

The Original Magic Wand
My desert island pick, this is incredibly versatile and durable.
https://www.vibratex.com

Silver Bullet
This battery-operated clitoral stimulator is cheap and easy to use, making it an excellent toy to try to help you figure out what kind of vibration you like.
https://calexotics.com/pocket-exotics-vibrating-silver-bullet-5-05-2-silver.html

Zumio
This is tiny but mighty and can produce orgasms in many people super quickly!
https://www.early2bed.com/zumio.html

Satisfyer Pro Plus Vibration
The Air Pulse technology is very different from the sensations from a vibrator, and the added "traditional" vibration from this toy gives it an extra dimension of fun.
https://us.satisfyer.com/us/products/air-pulse-technology/air-pulse-stimulators
-vibration/pro-2/

We-Vibe Melt

This uses Pleasure Air technology to stimulate the clitoris and has a low profile for using with a partner. It also can connect to your smartphone so your faraway lover can take over the controls.

https://www.early2bed.com/we-vibe-melt.html

We-Vibe Chorus

This is a vibe that you can wear during intercourse for a whole lot of sensation internally and externally at the same time. It can be used with a pressure-sensitive handheld remote or your smartphone!

https://www.we-vibe.com/us/chorus#color=26

We-Vibe Nova

One of the best dual-action toys on the market, this provides internal and external stimulation at the same time and has a bendable shaft for customization. Also works with your smartphone!

https://www.we-vibe.com/us/nova2

Max Link Silicone Cockring

A rechargeable vibrating cockring that provides hands-free clitoral stimulation during intercourse.

https://www.early2bed.com/max-silicone-cockring.html

Enchanted Rabbit

For those who want deep penetration with clitoral stimulation, this thrusting toy does all the work for you.

https://calexotics.com/enchanted-exciter-9-20-3-pink.html

Vision of Love Dildo

One of the cutest dildos I've seen, this is small enough for beginners and fits great in a dildo harness. The silicone is silky smooth to the touch.

https://www.early2bed.com/vision-of-love-dildo.html

Limba Flex Dildo

This thinner dildo has a malleable wire inside so you can decide what shape you want your toy to be, and then change your mind later.

https://us.funfactory.com/products/limba-flex

Graduate Glass Dildo

Glass is wonderful for putting pressure on the G-Spot or for people looking for less friction with thrusting.

https://www.early2bed.com/xr-brands-the-graduate-glass-dildo.html

Njoy Pure Wand

Everyone's favorite G-Spot toy, this heavy stainless wand is also great for experimenting with temperature play and is pretty enough to be a sculpture.

https://www.njoytoys.com/product/purewand/

The Mood Plug Trainer Kit

If you are looking to explore the backdoor, this graduated kit is a perfect way to get your body into new sensations gradually.

https://www.early2bed.com/mood-plug-trainer-kit.html

Notes

Chapter 1

1. Rahmat O. Raffi, Kamran S. Moghissi, Anthony G. Sacco, "Proteins of Human Vaginal Fluid," The American Fertility Society, December 1977, https://www.fertstert.org /article/S0015-0282(16)42982-1/pdf

2. Elena Shipitsyna, Annika Roos, Raluca Datcu, Anders Hallén, Hans Fredlund, S. Jørgen Jensen, Lars Engstrand, Magnus Unemo, "Composition of the Vaginal Microbiota in Women of Reproductive Age—Sensitive and Specific Molecular Diagnosis of Bacterial Vaginosis Is Possible?" U.S. National Library of Medicine, PLoS One, April 9, 2013, https://www.ncbi.nlm.nih.gov/pmc/articles/PMC3621988/

3. Marshall W., Tanner J. Puberty. In: Davis J., Dobbing J., editors. Scientific Foundations of Paediatrics. London: Heinemann; 1974.

Chapter 2

1. Stephen Quirke, "Kahun Medical Papyrus," Digital Egypt for Universities, University College London, 2002, https://www.ucl.ac.uk/museums-static/digitalegypt//med /birthpapyrus.html

2. https://scribalterror.blogs.com/scribal_terror/2006/05/aretaeus_of_cap.html

3. Erica Wright, "Magic to Heal the 'Wandering Womb' in Antiquity," #Folklore Thursday, January 18, 2018, https://folklorethursday.com/folklife /magic-to-heal-the-wandering-womb-in-antiquity/

4. JR Thorpe, "The Bizarre History of the Tampon," *Bustle*, November 19, 2015, https://www.bustle.com/articles/124929-the-history-of-the-tampon-because-they -havent-always-been-for-periods

5. Stephen Quirke, "Kahun Medical Papyrus," Digital Egypt for Universities, University College London, 2002, https://www.ucl.ac.uk/museums-static/digitalegypt//med /birthpapyrus.html

6. Izharul Hasan, Mohd Zulkifle, A.H. Ansari, A.M.K. Sherwani, Mohd Shakir, *History of Ancient Egyptian Obstetrics & Gynecology: A Review*, (Bangalore: Dept of Preventive and Social Medicine), 2017

7. Stevens, J.M. Medical Journal of Australia 2: 949-952, 1975. https://doi.org/10.5694 /j.1326-5377.1975.tb106465.x

8. John M. Riddle, *Contraception and Abortion from the Ancient World to the Renaissance*, (London: Harvard University Press), 1992

9. Dr. Kate Lister, "Victorian Doctors Were Not Using Vibrators on Female Patients—It Was Even Stranger Than That," *iNews*, Associated Newspapers Limited, November 12, 2018, https://inews.co.uk/opinion/comment/victorian-doctors-were-not-using-vibrators-on -female-patients-it-was-even-stranger-than-that-221027

10. Geri Walton, "Marie Boivin: A French Midwife and Doctor," Geri Walton, Rooster Press, May 15, 2017, https://www.geriwalton.com/french-midwife-and-doctor-named -marie-boivin/

Chapter 3

1. Mary Lewis, "Children Aren't Starting Puberty Younger, Medieval Skeletons Reveal," Phys.org, Science X Network, February 12, 2018, https://phys.org/news/2018-02 -children-puberty-younger-medieval-skeletons.html

2. Stuart Blackman, "Do Any Non-Human Animals Menstruate?" Discover Wildlife (from the team at BBC *Wildlife Magazine*), September 1, 2017, https://www.discoverwildlife.com /animal-facts/do-any-non-human-animals-menstruate/

3. Kathryn Clancy, "I Don't Have a 28-Day Menstrual Cycle, and Neither Should You," *Scientific American*, Nature America Inc., December 23, 2010, https://blogs .scientificamerican.com/guest-blog/i-dont-have-a-28-day-menstrual-cycle-and -neither-should-you/

4. Martha K. McClintock, "Menstrual Synchrony and Suppression," *Nature*, Springer Nature Limited, January 1971, https://www.nature.com/articles/229244a0

5. Luis Villazon, "Is it coincidental that the human menstrual cycle is about the same length as the Moon cycle?" Science Focus, *BBC Science Focus Magazine,* n.d., https://www.sciencefocus.com/the-human-body/is-it-coincidental-that-the -human-menstrual-cycle-is-about-the-same-length-as-the-moon-cycle/

6. Charlotte McDonald, "Is it true that periods synchronise when women live together?" *BBC News,* September 7, 2016, https://www.bbc.com/news/magazine-37256161

7. Anna Ziomkiewicz, "Menstrual synchrony: Fact or artifact?" *Polish Academy of Sciences,* December 2005, https://sites.oxy.edu/clint /physio/article/MenstrualsynchronyFactorartifact.pdf

8. Chris Knight, "Menstruation and the Origins of Culture," Radical Anthropology Group, University College London, 1987, http://radicalanthropologygroup.org/sites /default/files/pdf/pub_chris_thesis.pdf

9. Jen Bell, "What was it like to get your period in ancient Greece?" HelloClue, October 31, 2018, https://helloclue.com/articles/culture/what-was-it-like-to-get-your -period-in-ancient-greece

10. Kate Wheeling, "A Brief History of Menstrual Blood Myths," *Pacific Standard Magazine*, June 14, 2017, https://psmag.com/news/a-brief-history-of-menstrual-blood-myths

11. Pliny the Elder, *Natural History*, Loeb Classical Library, Harvard University Press, n.d., https://www.loebclassics.com/view/pliny_elder-natural_history/1938/pb_LCL352.549.xml

12. (Ernster, Lancet June 29, 1974, 1347). https://doi.org/10.1016/S0140-6736(74)90718-1

13. Siobahn Fenton, "Swimming pool bans women on their periods over 'contamination' concerns," *Independent*, August 11, 2016, https://www.independent.co.uk/news/world /asia/swimming-pool-accused-misogyny-after-banning-women-their-periods-over -contamination-concerns-a7184786.html

14. Siobhan Fenton, "Swimming Pool Bans Women on Their Periods Over 'Contamination' Concerns," *Independent*, August 2016, https://www.independent.co.uk/news/world/asia /swimming-pool-accused-of-misogyny-after-banning-women-on-their-periods -over-contamination-concerns-a7184786.html

15. Chris Knight, "Menstruation and the Origins of Culture," Radical Anthropology Group, University College London, 1987, http://radicalanthropologygroup.org/sites /default/files/pdf/pub_chris_thesis.pdf

16. M. Rezaeyan, P. Khedri, N. Abdali, Ashraf, D. Moghadam, "The impact of extra virgin olive oil on primary dysmenorrhea in comparison to the ibuprofen," Scholars Research Library, 2015, https://www.scholarsresearchlibrary.com/articles/the-impact-of-extra -virgin-olive-oil-on-primary-dysmenorrhea-in-comparison-to-the-ibuprofen.pdf

17. W.R. Phipps, M.C. Martini, J.W. Lampe, J.L. Slavin, M.S Kurzer, "Effect of flax seed ingestion on the menstrual cycle," National Library of Medicine, The Journal of Clinical Endocrinology and Metabolism, November 1993, https://pubmed.ncbi.nlm .nih.gov/8077314/

18. Mona Chalabi, "How Many Women Don't Use Tampons?" FiveThirtyEight, October 1, 2015, https://fivethirtyeight.com/features/how-many-women-dont-use-tampons/

19. Susan Dudley, Salwa Nassar, Emily Hartman, Sandy Wang, "Tampon Safety," National Center for Health Research, n.d., https://www.center4research.org/tampon-safety/

20. Maegan Boutot, "Toxic Shock Syndrome (TSS) and menstrual products: A short history," HelloClue, April 22, 2019, https://helloclue.com/articles/cycle-a-z/toxic-shock -syndrome-and-menstrual-products-a-short-history

21. Mary Bellis, "A Brief History of the Tampon," ThoughtCo, February 2020, thoughtco .com/history-of-the-tampon-4018968.

22. "Menstrual Care Products and Toxic Chemicals," Women's Voices for the Earth, n.d., https://www.womensvoices.org/menstrual-care-products/

23. Aayushi Pratap, "Periods still a taboo in Indian society: TISS study," Mumbai News, *Hindustan Times*, December 19, 2016, https://www.hindustantimes.com/mumbai -news/periods-still-a-taboo-in-indian-society-tiss-study/story -Dc5Muh2PWkJkbGg2j5DhWO.html

24. Jeffrey Gettleman, "Where a Taboo Is Leading to the Deaths of Young Girls," *New York Times*, June 19, 2018, https://www.nytimes.com/2018/06/19/world/asia/nepal -women-menstruation-period.html

25. Maride Espada, "Period Taboo Around the World," *TeenVogue*, Condé Nast, May 28, 2018, https://www.teenvogue.com/story/period-taboo-around-the-world; Anna Druet, "How did menstruation become taboo?" *Clued In*, Medium, September 8, 2017, https://medium.com/clued-in/how-did-menstruation-become-taboo-3c626585c87

26. The Menorrhagia Research Group, Gillian Warrilow, Caroline Kirkham, Khaled MK Ismail, Katrina Wyatt, Paul Dimmock, Shaughn O'Brien, "Quantification of menstrual blood loss," The Obstetrician & Gynaecologist, John Wiley & Sons Inc., January 24, 2011, https://obgyn.onlinelibrary.wiley.com/doi/pdf/10.1576/toag.6.2.88.26983

27. Olivia Petter, "More than half of women feel ashamed of their periods, finds survey," *Independent*, January 5, 2018, https://www.independent.co.uk/life-style/women-periods -ashamed-menstruation-half-survey-a8143416.html

Chapter 4

1. DeLee, Joseph B., A.M., M.D. *The Principles and Practice of Obstetrics.* 7th ed. (Philadelphia: W. B. Saunders Company, 1938) 319

2. https://www.theguardian.com/theguardian/2003/jun/26/features11.g2

3. Joyce Kong, "Pubic Hair Transplants Are a Thing in Korea," *Refinery29*, November 3, 2014, https://www.refinery29.com/en-us/pubic-hair-transplants

4. Jenn Sinrich, "What Is Vaginal Steaming?" Verywell Health, Dotdash, December 21, 2020, https://www.verywellhealth.com/vaginal-steaming-5087839

5. Debra Herbenick, Vanessa Schick, Michael Reece, Stephanie Sanders, and J. Dennis Fortenberry, "Pubic Hair Removal among Women in the United States: Prevalence, Methods, and Characteristics," The Journal of Sexual Medicine, Vol. 7, Issue 10, October 1, 2010, https://www.jsm.jsexmed.org/article/S1743-6095(15)32732-6/fulltext

Chapter 5

1. "Types of Human Papillomavirus," NYU Langone Health, n.d., https://nyulangone.org /conditions/human-papillomavirus-in-adults/types

Chapter 6

1. Jack D. Sobel, Caroline Mitchell, "Candida vulvovaginitis: Clinical manifestations and diagnosis," UpToDate, March 24, 2020, https://www.uptodate.com/contents /candida-vulvovaginitis-clinical-manifestations-and-diagnosis?search =candida%20vulvovaginitis%20clinical%20manifestations%20and%20diagnosis &source=search_result&selectedTitle=1~71&usage_type=default&display_rank=1

2. Elizabeth King, "Cracking Open the History of the Thong," *Vice*, February 9, 2016, https://www.vice.com/en/article/gvzabw/cracking-open-the-history-of-the-thong

3. "Vulvovaginal Candidiasis," Centers for Disease Control and Prevention, June 4, 2015, https://www.cdc.gov/std/tg2015/candidiasis.htm

4. Nalin Hetticarachchi, H. Ruth Ashbee, Janet D. Wilson, "Prevalence and management of non-albicans vaginal candidiasis," *Sexually Transmitted Infections*, BMJ Publishing Group, March 23, 2010, https://sti.bmj.com/content/86/2/99.info

5. Monica Helen Green, *The Trotula: A Medieval Compendium of Women's Medicine.* (Philadelphia: University of Pennsylvania Press, 2001), 76

6. Safaa Fares, Shadia Abd el Kader, Azza Ali Abd El Hamid, Hassan Mostaga Gaafar, "Effect of ingestion of yogurt containing *Lactobacillus acidophilus* on vulvovaginal candidiasis among women attending a gynecological clinic," *Egyptian Nursing Journal*, Wolters Kluwer, June 13, 2017, https://www.enj.eg.net/article.asp?issn =2090-6021;year=2017;volume=14;issue=1;spage=41;epage=49;aulast=Fares

7. M. Karaman, M. Bogavac, B. Radovanovic, J. Sudji, K Te Tešanović, L. Janjušević, "Origanum vulgare essential oil affects pathogens causing vaginal infections," *Journal of Applied Microbiology*, The Society for Applied Microbiology, February 7, 2017, https:// sfamjournals.onlinelibrary.wiley.com/doi/full/10.1111/jam.13413

8. Jennifer A. Shuford, James M. Steckelberg, Robin Patel, "Effects of Fresh Garlic Extract on *Candida albicans* Biofilms," Antimicrobial Agents and Chemotherapy, American Society of Microbiology, December 2004, https://aac.asm.org/content/49/1/473

9. D. O. Ogbolu, A. A. Oni, O. A. Daini, A. P. Oloko, "In vitro antimicrobial properties of coconut oil on *Candida* species in Ibadan, Nigeria," National Library of Medicine, Journal of Medicinal Food, June 2007, https://pubmed.ncbi.nlm.nih.gov/17651080/; Beena Shino, Faizal C. Peedikayil, Shyamala R. Jaiprakash, Gufran Ahmed Bijapur, Soni Kottayi, Deepak Jose, "Comparison of Antimicrobial Activity of Chlorhexidine, Coconut Oil, Probiotics, and Ketoconazole on *Candida albicans* Isolated in Children with Early Childhood Caries: An In Vitro Study," Hindawi, March 14, 2016, https:// www.hindawi.com/journals/scientifica/2016/7061587/

10. Judy Gopal, Vimala Anthonydhason, Manikandan Muthu, Enkhtaivan Gansukh, Somang Jung, Sechul Chul, Sivanesan Iyyakkannu, "Authenticating apple cider vinegar's home remedy claims: Antibacterial, Antifungal, antiviral properties and cytotoxcitiy aspect," *Natural Product Research*, Taylor & Francis Online, November 29, 2017, https://www .tandfonline.com/doi/citedby/10.1080/14786419.2017.1413567?scroll=top&needAccess=true

11. Alexander M. Maley, Jack L. Arbiser, "Gentian Violet: A 19th century drug re-emerges in the 21st century," Wiley Online Library, Experimental Dermatology, October 7, 2013, https://onlinelibrary.wiley.com/doi/full/10.1111/exd.12257

12. Maura Di Vito, Paola Mattarelli, Monica Modesto, Antonietta Girolamo, Milva Ballardini, Annunziata Tamburro, Marcello Meledandri, Francesca Mondello, "In Vitro Activity of Tea Tree Oil Vaginal Suppositories against Candida spp. and Probiotic Vaginal Microbiota," National Library of Medicine, Phytotherapy Research, October 29, 2015, https://pubmed.ncbi.nlm.nih.gov/26235937/

13. Andrew B. Shreiner, John Y. Kao, and Vincent B. Young, "The Gut Microbiome in Health and in Disease," Current Opinion in Gastroenterology, 31, no. 1, January 2015, https://journals.lww.com/co-gastroenterology/Abstract/2015/01000/The_gut _microbiome_in_health_and_in_disease.12.aspx

14. Jack D. Sobel, Caroline Mitchell, "Candida vulvovaginitis: Clinical manifestations and diagnosis," UpToDate, March 24, 2020, https://www.uptodate.com/contents/candida -vulvovaginitis-clinical-manifestations-and-diagnosis?search=candida%20vulvovaginitis %20clinical%20manifestations%20and%20diagnosis&source=search_result &selectedTitle=1~71&usage_type=default&display_rank=1

15. Ji-Yeong Im, Deok-Sang, Hwang, Jin-Moo Lee, Chang-Hoon, Lee, Jun-Bock Jang, "Research Trends of the Acupuncture Treatment for Vulvodynia," The Korean Journal of Obstetrics and Gynecology, February 22, 2019, https://www.koreascience.or.kr /article/JAKO201912262463422

16. "The low-oxalate diet," Vulval Pain Society, 2019, http://www.vulvalpainsociety.org /vps/index.php/treatments/the-low-oxalate-diet

17. Lynette J. Margesson, Hope K. Haefner, "Vulvar lesions: Differential diagnosis of vesicles, bullae, erosions, and ulcers," UpToDate, February 3, 2021, https://www .uptodate.com/contents/vulvar-lesions-differential-diagnosis-of-vesicles-bullae -erosions-and-ulcers; Susan Kellogg Spadt, Sheryl Kingsberg, "Treatment of vulvodynia (vulvar pain of unknown cause)," UpToDate, April 11, 2020, https://www.uptodate.com /contents/treatment-of-vulvodynia-vulvar-pain-of-unknown-cause?search=vulvodynia &source=search_result&selectedTitle=1~30&usage_type=default&display_rank =1#H155116773

18. Kate Lister, "Throwback Thursday: The long and surprising history of women using their genitals in cooking," *iNews*, Associated Newspapers Limited, July 6, 2017, https://inews.co.uk/essentials/long-surprising-history-women-using-genitals-cooking-77082

Chapter 7

1. Jack D. Sobel, Caroline Mitchell, "Bacterial vaginosis: Clinical manifestations and diagnosis," UpToDate, September 4, 2020, https://www.uptodate.com/contents/bacterial-vaginosis-clinical-manifestations-and-diagnosis?search=bacterial-vaginosis-clinical-manifestations-and-diagno-sis&source=search_result&selectedTitle=1~112&usage_type=default&display_rank=1
2. Alexis Record, "Vagina Power and the History of Christian Symbols," Patheos, November 30, 2016, https://www.patheos.com/blogs/removingthefigleaf/2016/11/vagina-power/

Chapter 8

1. Marissa Rhodes, "Underwear: A History of Intimate Apparel," Dig Podcast, June 24, 2018, https://digpodcast.org/2018/06/24/underwear-intimate-apparel
2. Thomas D'Urfey, "PUSS in a Corner," Early English Books Online Text Creation Partnership, n.d., https://quod.lib.umich.edu/e/eebo/A36960.0001.001/1:7?rgn=div1;view=fulltext
3. Thomas D'Urfey, *Wit and Mirth: Or Pills to Purge Melancholy*, (New York: Folklore Library Publishers, Inc, 1959), https://www.gutenberg.org/files/33404/33404-h/33404-h.htm
4. "Pussy," Online Etymology Dictionary, Douglas Harper, n.d., https://www.etymonline.com/word/pussy
5. "Pussy whipped," Dictionary.com, n.d., https://www.dictionary.com/e/slang/pussy-whipped/
6. Mina Moriarty, "A Brief History of the Cunt," *The Establishment*, Medium, February 9, 2018, https://medium.com/the-establishment/a-brief-history-of-the-cunt-a755b5df4a4
7. Deidre Mask, "How Did England Get Its Bizarro Street Names?" Literary Hub, April 9, 2020, https://lithub.com/how-did-england-get-its-bizarro-street-names/
8. Barbara G. Walker, *The Woman's Encyclopedia of Myths and Secrets*, (San Francisco: HarperOne, 1983), 197
9. Greg Polkosnik, "Ethel Merman," *Star Struck Style*, WordPress, January 16, 2017, https://gregpolkosnik.com/2017/01/16/ethel-merman/

Chapter 9

1. Jan L. Shifren, "Overview of sexual dysfunction in women: Management," UpToDate, July 16, 2020, https://www.uptodate.com/contents/overview-of-sexual-dysfunction-in-women-management#:~:text=In%20the%20United%20States%2C%20approximately, or%20a%20combination%20of%20these

2. Gwenyth Wren, "Orgasm equality is a long time coming," *The McGill Tribune*, SPT, October 23, 2018, http://www.mcgilltribune.com/sci-tech/orgasm-equality-is-a-long-time-coming-221018/#:~:text=In%20a%20recent%20study%20from,women%20could %20say%20the%20same

3. Richard Francis Burton, *The Kama Sutra and Ananga Ranga, with an Introduction by Anne Hardgrove* (Barnes & Noble, 2006), xviii

4. P. Cryle, A. Moore, *Frigidity, an Intellectual History*, (Palgrave Macmillan UK, 2011), 30

5. R. Syed, "Knowledge of the "Gräfenberg zone" and female ejaculation in ancient Indian sexual science. A medical history contribution," National Library of Medicine Sudhoffs Arch, 1999, https://pubmed.ncbi.nlm.nih.gov/10705806/

6. Beverly Whipple, "Ejaculation, female," Wiley Online Library, John Wiley & Sons, Inc., November 17, 2014, https://onlinelibrary.wiley.com/doi/full/10.1002/9781118896877 .wbiehs125; Zlatko Pastor, Roman Chmel, "Differential diagnostics of female 'sexual,' fluids: A narrative review," National Library of Medicine, International Urogynecology Journal, December 28, 2017, https://pubmed.ncbi.nlm.nih.gov/29285596/

7. E. Grafenberg, "The role of urethra in female orgasm," *International Journal of Sexology*, February 1950, http://www.andreadrian.de/Sex_und_Arbeitsteilung_Mann _Frau/1950_Graefenberg_The_Role_of_Urethra_in_Female_Orgasm.pdf

8. Rebecca Adams, "The G-Spot and 'Vaginal Orgasm' Are Myths, According to New Clinical Review," *HuffPost*, October 9, 2014, https://www.huffpost.com/entry/g-spot -vaginal-orgasm-myth_n_5947930

9. Carol Anderson Darling, J. Kenneth Davidson, Colleen Conway-Welch, "Female ejaculation: Perceived origins, the Grafenberg spot/area, and sexual responsiveness," SpringerLink, *Springer Nature*, February 1990, https://link.springer.com/article /10.1007/BF01541824

10. Ibid

11. Clayton English, Anne Muhleisen, Jose A. Rey, "Flibanserin (Addyi) The First FDA-Approved Treatment for Female Sexual Interest/Arousal Disorder in Premenopausal Women," U.S. National Library of Medicine, Pharmacy & Therapeutics Journal, April 2017, https://www.ncbi.nlm.nih.gov/pmc/articles/PMC5358680/; "Clinical Trials Addyi Is Proven Safe and Effective," Addyi.com, Sprout Pharmaceuticals, n.d., https: //addyihcp.com/clinical-trials/

12. Sheryl A. Kingsberg, Anita H. Clayton, David Portman, Laura A. Williams, Julie Krop, Robert Jordan, Johna Lucas, James A. Simon, "Bremelanotide for the Treatment of Hypoactive Sexual Desire Disorder," Obstetrics & Gynecology, November 2019, https://journals.lww.com/greenjournal/Fulltext/2019/11000/Bremelanotide_for_the _Treatment_of_Hypoactive.2.aspx

13. Laura S. Leddy, Claire C. Yang, Bronwyn G. Stuckey, Maria Sudworth, Scott Haughie, Stefan Sultana, Kenneth R. Maravilla, "Influence of sildenafil on genital engorgement in women with female sexual arousal disorder," National Library of Medicine, *The Journal of Sexual Medicine*, May 23, 2012, https://pubmed.ncbi.nlm.nih.gov/22620487/

14. Charles Runels, Hugh Melnick, Ernest Debourbon, Lisbeth Roy, "A Pilot Study of the Effect of Localized Injection of Autologuous Platelet Rich Plasma (PRP) for the Treatment of Female Sexual Dysfunction," *Journal of Women's Health Care*, 2014, https://www.longdom.org/open-access/a-pilot-study-of-the-effect-of-localized -injections-of-autologous-platelet-rich-plasma-prp-for-the-treatment-of-female -sexual-dysfunction-2167-0420.1000169.pdf

15. https://my.clevelandclinic.org/health/treatments/17761-energy-based treatments -and-vaginal-rejuvenation

16. The North American Menopause Society, "Laser therapy gains credibility as effective option for treating vaginal problems," Science News, October 2, 2019, https://www .sciencedaily.com/releases/2019/10/191002112620.htm

17. Michael Krychman, Christopher G. Rowan, Bruce B. Allan, Leonard DeRogatis, Scott Durbin, Ashley Yacoubian, Deborah Wilkerson, "Effect of Single Treatment, Surface-Cooled Radiofrequency Therapy on Vaginal Laxity and Female Sexual Function: The VIVEVE I Randomized Controlled Trial," ScienceDirect, *The Journal of Sexual Medicine*, February 2017, https://www.sciencedirect.com/science/article/abs/pii /S1743609516308530

18. "Clinical Research," GainsWave, n.d., https://gainswave.com/clinical-research/

19. W. Everaerd, J. Dekker, "Treatment of secondary orgasmic dysfunction: A comparison of systematic desensitization and sex therapy," National Library of Medicine, Behaviour Research and Therapy, 1982, https://pubmed.ncbi.nlm.nih.gov/6124236/

20. Masters, W., & Johnson, V. E., *Human Sexual Inadequacy*, (New York: Little, Brown and Company, 1970); Weiner, L., & Avery-Clark, C., *Sensate Focus: Clarifying the Masters and Johnson's Model. Sexual and Relationship Therapy*, 2014, n.d., http://www .sextherapiststlouis.com/files/SensateFocusOnly.pdf

21. Naomi Williamson, "16 Bizarre Aphrodisiacs Throughout History," *Woman's Day*, Hearst Magazine Media, Inc., March 11, 2015, https://www.womansday.com/relationships/sex -tips/g1775/bizarre-aphrodisiacs-throughout-history/?slide=16

22. Christopher Kemp, "An Excerpt from Floating Gold: A Natural (and Unnatural) History of Ambergris," The University of Chicago Press Books, University of Chicago Press, April 6, 2012, https://press.uchicago.edu/books/excerpt/2012/kemp_floating .html; S.A. Taha, M.W. Islam, A.M. Ageel, "Effect of ambrein, a major constituent of ambergris, on masculine sexual behavior in rats," National Library of Medicine, Archives internationales de pharmacodynamie et de thérapie, March 1995, https: //pubmed.ncbi.nlm.nih.gov/8540767/

23. "Can food fire up your love life?" Kencko, n.d., https://www.kencko.com/blogs/the-goods /can-food-fire-up-your-love-life

24. Alexandra Malmed, "Love Potions: A Brief History of Aphrodisiacs," Vogue, Condé Nast, February 11, 2017, https://www.vogue.com/article/what-foods-are-aphrodisiacs-history

25. "Sexual Response Cycle," Cleveland Clinic, March 8, 2021, https://my.clevelandclinic .org/health/articles/9119-sexual-response-cycle

26. Joseph Stromberg, "This is what your brain looks like during an orgasm," Vox, Vox Media, April 1, 2015, https://www.vox.com/2015/4/1/8325483/orgasms-science

27. Ibid.

28. Suzannah Weiss, "Your Most Common Questions About the Female Orgasm, Answered," Glamour, Condé Nast, February 26, 2019, https://www.glamour.com/story /the-most-common-questions-about-the-female-orgasm-answered

29. E.O. Laumann, A. Nicolosi, D.B. Glasser, A. Paik, C. Gingell, E. Moreira, T. Wang, "Sexual Problems among Women and Men Aged 40–80 y: Prevalence and Correlates Identified in the Study of Sexual Attitudes and Behaviors," National Library of Medi-cine, International Journal of Impotence Research, January 2005, https://pubmed .ncbi.nlm.nih.gov/15215881/; Laurie Mintz, "The Orgasm Gap: Simple Truth & Sexual Solutions," Psychology Today, October 4, 2015, https://www.psychologytoday.com/us/ blog/stress-and-sex/201510/the-orgasm-gap-simple-truth-sexual-solutions

30. Diane Kelly, "9 Animals That Masturbate (Other Than Humans)", Gizmodo, August 12, 2015, https://gizmodo.com/9-animals-that-masturbate-other-than-humans-1723592357

Chapter 10

1. James Sorensen, Katherine E. Bautista, Georgine Lamvu, Jessica Feranec, "Evaluation and Treatment of Female Sexual Pain: A Clinical Review," U.S. National Library of Medicine, Cureus, March 2018, https://www.ncbi.nlm.nih.gov/pmc/articles/PMC5969816/

2. Marie-Andrée Lahaie, Stéphanie C. Boyer, Rhonda Amsel, Samir Khalifé, M. Yitzchak Binik, "Vaginismus: A Review of the Literature on the Classification/Diagnosis, Etiology, and Treatment," Sage Journals, Sage Publications Ltd, September 1, 2010, https://journals.sagepub.com/doi/full/10.2217/WHE.10.46

3. "Female genital mutilation," World Health Organization, February 3, 2020, https://www.who.int/news-room/fact-sheets/detail/female-genital-mutilation

4. "Female Genital Mutilation/Cutting (FGM/C)," Centers for Disease Control and Prevention, May 11, 2020, https://www.cdc.gov/reproductivehealth/womensrh/female-genital-mutilation.html

5. E. Sheehan, "Victorian clitoridectomy, Isaac Baker Brown and his harmless operative procedure," National Library of Medicine, Medical Anthropology Newsletter, August 1981, https://pubmed.ncbi.nlm.nih.gov/12263443/

6. Nawal M. Nour, "Female genital cutting: Clinical and cultural guidelines," National Library of Medicine, Obstetrical and Gynecological Survey, April 2004, https://pubmed.ncbi.nlm.nih.gov/15024227/

7. Jayant Pai Dhungat, "Female Genital Mutilation," National Library of Medicine, The Journal of the Association of Physicians of India, April 2019, https://pubmed.ncbi.nlm.nih.gov/31299853/; Lili Loofbourow, "The female price of male pleasure," *The Week*, January 25, 2018, https://theweek.com/articles/749978/female-price-male-pleasure

Chapter 11

1. Natalie Gil, "My Vagina Split": Keira Knightley Openly Discusses Her Childbirth in New Essay," *Refinery29*, Vice Media Group, October 5, 2018, https://www.refinery29.com/en-gb/2018/10/213194/keira-knightley-birth-feminism-essay

2. James E. Gleichert, "Etienne Joseph Jacquemin, Discoverer of 'Chadwick Sign,'" Journal of History of Medicine and Allied Sciences, Volume 26, No. 1, January 1971, Pages 75–80, https://academic.oup.com/jhmas/article-abstract/XXVI/1/75/681229?redirectedFrom=fulltext

3. Graham P. Stafford, Jennifer L. Parker, Emmanuel Amabebe, James Kistler, Steven Reynolds, Victoria Stern, Martyn Paley, Dilly O.C. Anumba, "Spontaneous Preterm Birth Is Associated with Differential Expression of Vaginal Metabolites by Lactobacilli-Dominated Microflora," U.S. National Library of Medicine, Frontiers in Physiology, August 23, 2017, https://www.ncbi.nlm.nih.gov/pmc/articles/PMC5572350/

4. Victoria L. Handa, "Effect of Pregnancy and Childbirth on Urinary Incontinence and Pelvic Organ Prolapse," UpToDate, March 9 2020, https://www.uptodate.com/contents/effect-of-pregnancy-and-childbirth-on-urinary-incontinence-and-pelvic-organ-prolapse?search=effect%20of%20pregnancy%20and%20childbirth%20on%20urinary%20incontinence%20and%20site%20specific%20repair%20of%20pelvic%20organ%20prolapse%20pro%20olapse&source=search_result&selectedTitle=1~150&usage_type=default&display_rank=1

5. Ibid.

6. Elizabeth A. Frankman, Li Wang, Clareann H. Bunker, Jerry L. Lowder, "Episiotomy in the United States: Has anything changed?" National Library of Medicine, American Journal of Obstetrics and Gynecology, May 2009, https://pubmed.ncbi.nlm.nih.gov /19243733/

7. T. Postel, "Childbirth climax: The revealing of obstetrical orgasm," Science Direct, Sexologies, October 2013, https://www.sciencedirect.com/science/article/abs/pii /S1158136013000467?via%3Dihub

8. Rebecca G. Rogers, Noelle Borders, Lawrence M. Leeman, and Leah L. Albers, "Does Spontaneous Genital Tract Trauma Impact Postpartum Sexual Function?" J Midwifery Women's Health, 2009 54 (2): 98–103, https://www.ncbi.nlm.nih.gov/pmc/ articles/PMC2730880/

9. "Heaviest birth," Guinness World Records, n.d., https://www.guinnessworldrecords .com/world-records/heaviest-birth

Chapter 12

1. The Aesthetic Society, "Aesthetic Plastic Surgery National Databank, Statistics," The Aesthetic Society, 2019, https://www.surgery.org/sites/default/files/Aesthetic-Society _Stats2019Book_FINAL.pdf

2. Darryl J. Hodgkinson, Glen Hait, "Aesthetic vaginal labioplasty," National Library of Medicine, Plastic and Reconstructive Surgery, September 1984, https://pubmed.ncbi .nlm.nih.gov/6473559/

3. Placik OJ, Arkins JP, "Plastic surgery trends parallel Playboy magazine: The pudenda preoccupation," National Library of Medicine, Aesthetic Surgery Journal, September 2014, https://pubmed.ncbi.nlm.nih.gov/25168807/; The Aesthetic Society, "New Data from The Aesthetic Society Indicates Decrease in Breast Augmentation Surgery," Cision PR Newswire, May 19, 2020, https://www.prnewswire.com/news-releases/new -data-from-the-aesthetic-society-indicates-decrease-in-breast-augmentation-surgery -301061348.html#:~:text=The%20latest%20data%20illustrates%20a,(explantation) %20increased%2034.4%25.

4. "The Power of Female Sex," IMDB, n.d., https://www.imdb.com/title/tt0698688/

5. "Changing female body image through art," The Great Wall of Vagina, n.d., http://www.greatwallofvagina.co.uk/home

6. Zahra Barnes, "The Size of Your Vagina: Is It Normal?" *Women's Health*, Hearst Magazine Media, Inc., December 16, 2014, https://www.womenshealthmag.com/health /a19909228/vagina-size/

7. A. Kreklau, I. Vâz, F. Oehme, F. Strub, R. Brechbühl, C. Christmann, A. Günthert, "Measurement of a 'normal vulva' in women aged 15–84: A cross-sectional prospective single-centre study," Obstetrics & Gynaecology, An International Journal of Obstetrics and Gynaecology, June 25, 2018, https://obgyn.onlinelibrary.wiley.com/doi/full/10.1111 /1471-0528.15387

8. D. Veale, E. Eshkevari, N. Ellison, A. Costa, D. Robinson, A. Kavouni, L. Cardozo, "Psychological characteristics and motivation of women seeking labiaplasty," National Library of Medicine, Psychological Medicine, February 2014, https://pubmed.ncbi.nlm .nih.gov/23659496/

9. Saba Motakef, Jose Rodriguez-Feliz, Michael Chung, Michael Ingargiola, Victor Wong, Ashit Patel, "Vaginal Labiaplasty: Current Practices and a Simplified Classification System for Labial Protrusion," National Library of Medicine, Plastic and Reconstruction Surgery, March 2015, https://pubmed.ncbi.nlm.nih.gov/25719696/

Chapter 13

1. Penn & Teller: Bullshit!, "Abstinence" [4.10], 5 June 2006—Masturbation

2. John Kelly, "Shakespeare's dildo, and other secret Early Modern pleasures," *Strong Language*, WordPress, January 20, 2017, https://stronglang.wordpress.com/2017/01/20 /shakespeares-dildo-and-other-secret-early-modern-pleasures/

3. John Coulthart, "The Choise of Valentines, Or the Merie Ballad of Nash His Dildo," *feuilleton*, WordPress, http://www.johncoulthart.com/feuilleton/2011/02/14/the-choise -of-valentines-or-the-merie-ballad-of-nash-his-dildo/

4. Rachael Redjou, "Shunga, Erotic Art in the Tokugawa Era," Cedar, Western Washington University, 2016, https://cedar.wwu.edu/library_researchaward/10/

5. Robinson Meyer, Ashley Fetters, "Victorian-Era Orgasms and the Crisis of Peer Review," *The Atlantic*, September 6, 2018, https://www.theatlantic.com/health/archive /2018/09/victorian-vibrators-orgasms-doctors/569446/; Hallie Lieberman, *Buzz: The Stimulating History of the Sex Toy*, (New York: Pegasus Press, 2017)

6. Janet Burns, "How the 'Niche' Sex Toy Market Grew into an Unstoppable $15B Industry," *Forbes*, July 15, 2016, https://www.forbes.com/sites/janetwburns/2016/07/15 /adult-expo-founders-talk-15b-sex-toy-industry-after-20-years-in-the-fray/?sh=- 9227c5a5bb95

7. Fergus Linnane, *London: The Wicked City: A Thousand Years of Vice in the Capital*, (London: Robson Press, 2003)

8. Statista Research Department, "Size of the sex toy market worldwide 2019–2026," Statista, Statista Research Department, November 30, 2020, https://www.statista.com /statistics/587109/size-of-the-global-sex-toy-market/

9. Ayo Osobamiro, "6 TV Shows That Helped Normalize Female Masturbation," Femestella, April 18, 2020, http://www.femestella.com/6-tv-shows-normalize-female -masturbation/; Mehera Bonner, "In the Name of Feminism, 28 Movies and TV Shows That Feature Female Masturbation," *Marie Claire*, Hearst Digital Media, June 8, 2019, https://www.marieclaire.com/celebrity/news/g4850/best-masturbation-scenes/

Chapter 14

1. Barbara G. Walker, *The Woman's Encyclopedia of Myths and Secrets*, (San Francisco: HarperOne, 1983), 641

2. T. Igancio Montoya, P. Antonio Maldonado, Jesus F. Acevedo, R. Ann Word, "Effect of Vaginal or Systemic Estrogen on Dynamics of Collagen Assembly in the Rat Vaginal Wall," U.S. National Library of Medicine, Biology of Reproduction, December 23, 2014, https://www.ncbi.nlm.nih.gov/pmc/articles/PMC4326728/#:~:text=The%20vaginal %20wall%20is%20made,vaginal%20wall%20is%20poorly%20understood

3. Fernand Labrie, David Archer, Céline Bouchard, Michel Fortier, Leonello Cusan, José-Luis Gomez, Ginette Girard, Mira Baron, Normand Ayotte, Michèle Moreau, Robert Dubé, Isabelle Côté, Claude Labrie, Lyne Lavoie, Louise Berger, Lucy Gilbert, Céline Martel, John Balser, "Effect of intravaginal dehydroepiandrosterone (Prasterone) on libido and sexual dysfunction in postmenopausal women," National Library of Medicine, Menopause, October 2009, https://pubmed.ncbi.nlm.nih.gov/19424093/

4. S. Abbas Shobeiri, M.H. Kerkhof, Vatche A. Minassian, Tony Bazi, "IUGA committee opinion: Laser-based vaginal devices for treatment of stress urinary incontinence, genitourinary syndrome of menopause, and vaginal laxity," International Urogynecology Journal, September 14, 2018, https://www.iuga.org/index.php?preview=1&option =com_dropfiles&format=&task=frontfile.download&catid=103&id=74&Itemid =1000000000000

5. Lloyd, Elisabeth Anne, *The Case of the Female Orgasm: Bias in the Science of Evolution*, (Cambridge: Harvard University Press, 2009), 53

6. S. Cavkaytar, M.K. Kokanali, H.O. Topcu, O.S. Aksakal, M. Doganay, "Effect of home-based Kegel exercises on quality of life in women with stress and mixed urinary incontinence," Taylor & Francis Online, Journal of Obstetrics and Gynaecology, September 29, 2014, https://www.tandfonline.com/doi/abs/10.3109/01443615.2014.9 60831; Soheila Nazarpour, Masoumeh Simbar, Fahimeh Ramezani Tehrani, Hamid Alavi Majd, "Effects of Sex Education and Kegel Exercises on the Sexual Function of Postmenopausal Women: A Randomized Clinical Trial," ScienceDirect, The Journal Sexual Medicine, July 2017, https://www.sciencedirect.com/science/article/abs/pii/ S174360951731192X

7. Meghan Rabbitt, "Doing Kegels But Not Noticing a Difference? These 5 Simple Yoga Poses Can Help," *Prevention*, Hearst Magazine Media, September 7, 2017, https://www .prevention.com/sex/a20489811/yoga-and-kegels-for-strong-pelvic-floor/

Chapter 15

1. J Marion Sims, *The Story of My Life*, ed. H. Marion Sims, (New York: D. Appleton and Company, 1886), 231

2. Verrie Elwin, "The Vagina Dentata Legend," The British Psychological Society, British Journal of Medical Psychology, June 1943, https://bpspsychub.onlinelibrary.wiley.com /doi/abs/10.1111/j.2044-8341.1943.tb00338.x

3. Barbara G. Walker, *The Woman's Encyclopedia of Myths and Secrets*, (San Francisco: HarperOne, 1983), 1035

4. Justin Ling, "Incels Are Radicalized and Dangerous. But Are They Terrorists?" *FP*, The Slate Group, June 2, 2020, https://foreignpolicy.com/2020/06/02/incels-toronto-attack -terrorism-ideological-violence/

5. Kelly Vance, "Deadly in Pink," East Bay Express, Weeklys, January 23, 2008, https://eastbayexpress.com/deadly-in-pink-1/

6. Michelle A. Gohr, "Do I Have Something in My Teeth? Vagina Dentata and Its Mani-festations within Popular Culture," Springer Link, *The Moral Panics of Sexuality*, 2013, https://doi.org/10.1057/9781137353177_2; Lauren Wissot, "Bite Me: *Teeth*," Slant Magazine, January 18, 2008, https://www.slantmagazine.com/film/bite-me-teeth/

7. P.B. Pendergrass, C.A. Reeves, M.W. Belovicz, D.J. Molter, J.H. White, "Comparison of vaginal shapes in Afro-American, Caucasian, and Hispanic women as seen with vinyl polysiloxane casting," National Library of Medicine, Gynecologic and Obstetric Investigation, 2000, https://pubmed.ncbi.nlm.nih.gov/10895030/; Kurt T. Barnhart, Adriana Izquierdo, E. Scott Pretorius, David M. Shera, Mayadah Shabbout, Alka Shaunik, "Baseline dimensions of the human vagina," Oxford Academic, Human Reproduction, June 2006, https://academic.oup.com/humrep/article/21/6/1618/724374

8. Rebecca G. Rogers, Tola B. Fashokun, "Pelvic organ prolapse in women: Epidemiology, risk factors, clinical manifestations, and management," UpToDate, February 11, 2020, https://www.uptodate.com/contents/pelvic-organ-prolapse-in-women-epidemiology -risk-factors-clinical-manifestations-and-management?search=cystocele&source =search_result&selectedTitle=1~45&usage_type=default&display_rank=1

9. *FeministMiranda*, "Sarah Baartman Saartjie," *FeministMiranda*, WordPress, February 4, 2019, https://myfeminism217659050.wordpress.com/2019/02/04/sarah-baartman -saartjie/; Caroline Elkins, "A Life Exposed," *New York Times*, January 14, 2007, https:// www.nytimes.com/2007/01/14/books/review/Elkins.t.html

10. Victoria L. Handa, Mark E. Lockhart, Julia R. Fielding, Catherine S. Bradley, Linda Brubakery, Geoffrey W. Cundiffy, Wen Ye, Holly E. Richter, "Racial Differences in Pelvic Anatomy by Magnetic Resonance Imaging," U.S. National Library of Medicine, HHS Public Access, April 2008, https://www.ncbi.nlm.nih.gov/pmc/articles/PMC2593128/

11. Janice A. Sabin, "How we fail black patients in pain," AAMC, January 6, 2020, https://www.aamc.org/news-insights/how-we-fail-black-patients-pain

12. Dorothy E. Roberts, "Race and the New Reproduction," *In Killing the Black Body: Race, Reproduction, and the Meaning of Liberty*, (New York: Vintage Books, a division of Penguin Random House LLC, 2017), 255; Bob Kronemyer, "How race/ethnicity influences endometriosis," Contemporary OB/GYN, May 22, 2019, https://www.contemporaryobgyn.net/view/how-raceethnicity-influences-endometriosis

13. Kelly M. Hoffman, Sophie Trawalter, Jordan R. Axt, M. Norman Oliver, "Racial bias in pain assessment and treatment recommendations, and false beliefs about biological differences between blacks and whites," U.S. National Library of Medicine, PNAS, April 19, 2016, https://www.ncbi.nlm.nih.gov/pmc/articles/PMC4843483/

14. Vidya Rao, "'You are not listening to me': Black women on pain and implicit bias in medicine," *Today*, NBC Universal, July 27, 2020, https://www.today.com/health/implicit-bias-medicine-how-it-hurts-black-women-t187866

15. Dr. David Pilgrim, "The Sapphire Caricature," Jim Crow Museum of Racist Memorabilia, Ferris State University, August 2008, https://www.ferris.edu/HTMLS/news/jimcrow/antiblack/sapphire.htm

16. http://www.newsweek-com.cdn.ampproject.org, 2008 campaign speech

17. Gene Demby, "The Truth Behind the Life of the Original 'Welfare-Queen'," Code Switch, NPR, December 20, 2013, https://www.npr.org/sections/codeswitch/2013/12/20/255819681/the-truth-behind-the-lies-of-the-original-welfare-queen

18. Rebecca Epstein, Jamilia J. Blake, Thalia González, *Girlhood Interrupted: The Erasure of Black Girls' Childhood*, Center on Poverty and Inequality, Georgetown Law, n.d., https://genderjusticeandopportunity.georgetown.edu/wp-content/uploads/2020/06/girlhood-interrupted.pdf; The Annie E. Casey Foundation, "New Study: The 'Adultification' of Black Girls," The Annie E. Casey Foundation, July 26, 2017, https://www.aecf.org/blog/new-study-the-adultification-of-black-girls/

19. Dr. David Pilgrim, "The Sapphire Caricature," Jim Crow Museum of Racist Memorabilia, Ferris State University, August 2008, https://www.ferris.edu/HTMLS/news/jimcrow/antiblack/sapphire.htm; Dr. David Pilgrim, "The Jezebel Stereotype," Jim Crown Museum of Racist Memorabilia, Ferris State University, July 2002, https://www.ferris.edu/jimcrow/jezebel/

20. Robert Beatty, "A Letter to Oprah: Thank You for Being the Nation's Super Mammy," *South Florida Times*, December 30, 2010, http://www.sfltimes.com/uncategorized /a-letter-to-oprah-thank-you-for-being-the-nations-super-mammy

21. Jennifer Harris, Elwood Watson, *The Oprah Phenomenon*, (Kentucky: University Press of Kentucky, 2007)

Index

About the Author

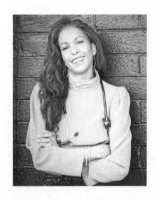

DR. NICOLE WILLIAMS is a native of East St. Louis, Illinois, and is a Board-certified obstetrician and gynecologist. With the philosophy of marrying both alternative and traditional medicine, Dr. Williams opened The Gynecology Institute of Chicago (GIC) in July 2013. Since that time, she has expanded the GIC to 3 locations and has cared for thousands of patients (and their vaginas). Dr. Williams has degrees in English Literature and Biochemistry from the University of Illinois at Urbana-Champaign and earned an MD from Loyola University Chicago.

In 2008, she made it to the final round of ABC's "The Mole" reality show, taking second place. Dr. Williams has appeared in *Cosmopolitan*, *Redbook*, *Prevention*, *Chicago Sun-Times*, *Women's Health*, Buzzfeed.com, *InStyle*, and *Bustle*. She is a tireless advocate for women's health issues, especially maternal issues, and has successfully lobbied Congress with the American College of Obstetricians and Gynecologists on behalf of her patients, having her formal remarks entered into the public record.

Dr. Williams also travels the world extensively, educating and operating on women who need it through various aid organizations—Haiti, Rwanda, Ghana, the Philippines, and Cambodia, to name just a few of these remote places. A dedicated teacher, she often takes a physician-in-training on these journeys to expand their global view. Dr. Williams has also made many appearances on ABC, NPR, WGN, CBS, and FOX Chicago as a noted speaker on women's health. In *This Is How You Vagina*, Dr. Williams seeks to dispel all the myths she still hears from patients every day about their vaginas and to empower them with vagina knowledge. She lives in Chicago, Illinois.